Wound Care
at a Glance

This title is also available as an e-book.
For more details, please see
www.wiley.com/buy/9781119590507
or scan this QR code:

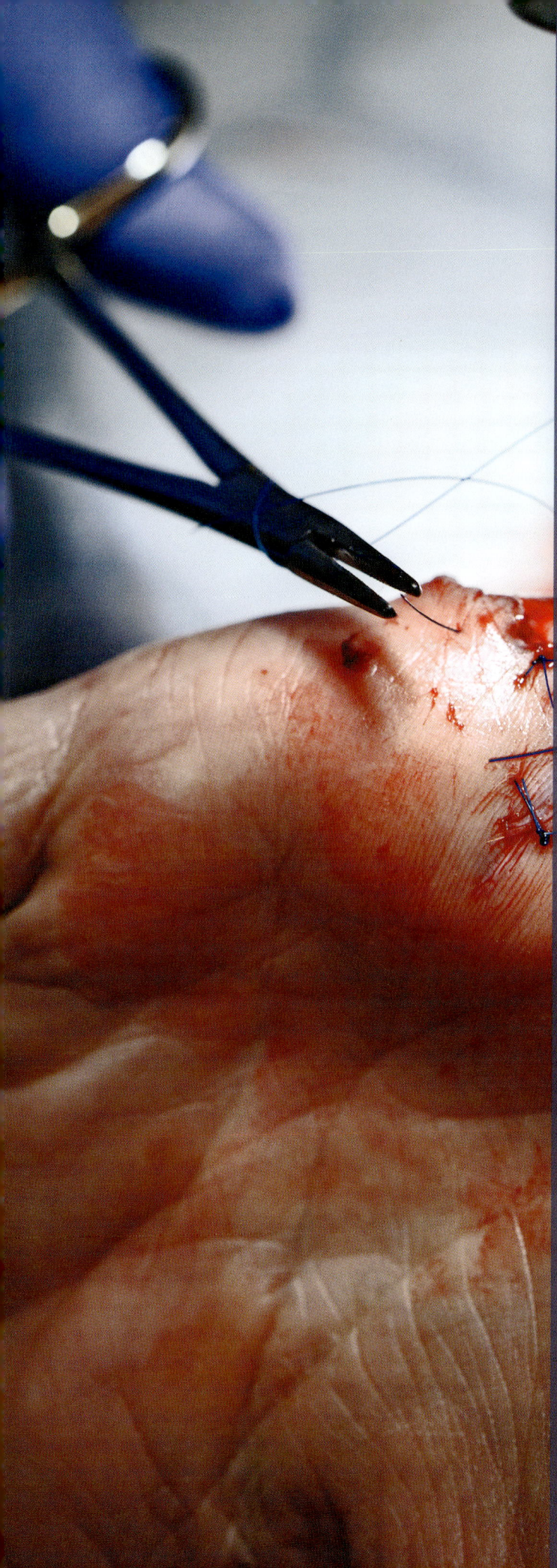

Wound Care at a Glance

Second Edition

Ian Peate
OBE FRCN
Head of School
School of Health Studies
Gibraltar Health Authority, Gibraltar;
Visiting Professor, St George's University
University of London and Kingston University
London, UK

Dr Melanie Stephens
PhD
Senior Lecturer in Adult Nursing
Lead for Interprofessional Education
Module Lead for Tissue Viability and Leg Ulcer
Management Modules
School of Health and Society
University of Salford
England, UK

Series Editor: Ian Peate

WILEY Blackwell

This edition first published 2020
© 2020 John Wiley & Sons Ltd

Edition History
John Wiley and Sons (1e, 2015)

All rights reserved. No part of this publication may be reproduced, stored in a retrieval system, or transmitted, in any form or by any means, electronic, mechanical, photocopying, recording or otherwise, except as permitted by law. Advice on how to obtain permission to reuse material from this title is available at http://www.wiley.com/go/permissions.

The right of Ian Peate and Melanie Stephens to be identified as the author(s) of this work has been asserted in accordance with law.

Registered Office(s)
John Wiley & Sons, Inc., 111 River Street, Hoboken, NJ 07030, USA
John Wiley & Sons Ltd, The Atrium, Southern Gate, Chichester, West Sussex, PO19 8SQ, UK

Editorial Office
9600 Garsington Road, Oxford, OX4 2DQ, UK

For details of our global editorial offices, customer services, and more information about Wiley products visit us at www.wiley.com.

Wiley also publishes its books in a variety of electronic formats and by print-on-demand. Some content that appears in standard print versions of this book may not be available in other formats.

Limit of Liability/Disclaimer of Warranty
The contents of this work are intended to further general scientific research, understanding, and discussion only and are not intended and should not be relied upon as recommending or promoting scientific method, diagnosis, or treatment by physicians for any particular patient. In view of ongoing research, equipment modifications, changes in governmental regulations, and the constant flow of information relating to the use of medicines, equipment, and devices, the reader is urged to review and evaluate the information provided in the package insert or instructions for each medicine, equipment, or device for, among other things, any changes in the instructions or indication of usage and for added warnings and precautions. While the publisher and authors have used their best efforts in preparing this work, they make no representations or warranties with respect to the accuracy or completeness of the contents of this work and specifically disclaim all warranties, including without limitation any implied warranties of merchantability or fitness for a particular purpose. No warranty may be created or extended by sales representatives, written sales materials or promotional statements for this work. The fact that an organization, website, or product is referred to in this work as a citation and/or potential source of further information does not mean that the publisher and authors endorse the information or services the organization, website, or product may provide or recommendations it may make. This work is sold with the understanding that the publisher is not engaged in rendering professional services. The advice and strategies contained herein may not be suitable for your situation. You should consult with a specialist where appropriate. Further, readers should be aware that websites listed in this work may have changed or disappeared between when this work was written and when it is read. Neither the publisher nor authors shall be liable for any loss of profit or any other commercial damages, including but not limited to special, incidental, consequential, or other damages.

Library of Congress Cataloging-in-Publication Data

Names: Peate, Ian, author. | Stephens, Melanie, author.
Title: Wound care at a glance / Ian Peate, Melanie Stephens.
Other titles: At a glance series (Oxford, England).
Description: Second edition. | Hoboken, NJ : Wiley Blackwell, 2020. | Series: At a glance series | Includes bibliographical references and index.
Identifiers: LCCN 2019034343 (print) | LCCN 2019034344 (ebook) | ISBN 9781119590507 (paperback) | ISBN 9781119590484 (adobe pdf) | ISBN 9781119590590 (epub)
Subjects: MESH: Wound Healing | Wounds and Injuries | Handbook
Classification: LCC RD93 (print) | LCC RD93 (ebook) | NLM WO 39 | DDC 617.1–dc23
LC record available at https://lccn.loc.gov/2019034343
LC ebook record available at https://lccn.loc.gov/2019034344

Cover Design: Wiley
Cover Image: © Johner Images/Getty Images

Set in 9.5/11.5pt Minion Pro by SPi Global, Pondicherry, India
Printed and bound in Singapore by Markono Print Media Pte Ltd

10 9 8 7 6 5 4 3 2 1

Contents

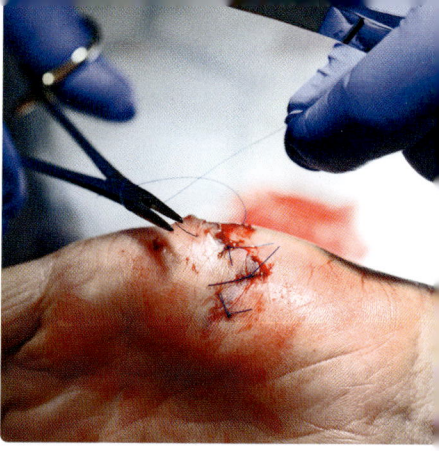

Preface to the second edition vii
Acknowledgements viii
How to use your textbook ix
About the companion website xi

Part 1 — Anatomy and physiology 1

1. The history of wound care 2
2. Anatomy and physiology of the skin 4
3. Psychological and social aspects of the skin 6
4. Body image 8
5. The skin and ageing 12

Part 2 — The normal healing process: acute wounds 15

6. Haemostasis 16
7. Inflammation 18
8. Proliferation (granulation and epithelialisation) 20
9. Maturation 22
10. Factors affecting wound-healing 24

Part 3 — The abnormal healing process: chronic wound healing 27

11. The impaired healing process 28
12. Factors affecting wound-healing 30
13. Nutrition and wound-healing 32
14. Incontinence and wounds 34
15. Vascular disease 36

Part 4 — Wound management in practice 39

16. Assessment of skin 40
17. Assessment of the patient with a wound 42
18. Classification of wounds 46
19. Legal and ethical aspects of wound care 48
20. Documenting wounds and keeping records 50
21. Evidence-based practice 52
22. Treatment options 54
23. Pain management 56

Part 5 Dressing selection 59

- **24** Principles of wound management I 60
- **25** Principles of wound management II 61
- **26** Managing wound exudate: moist wound healing, hydration and maceration 62
- **27** Generic wound products: mode of action 64
- **28** Choosing a wound care product 68
- **29** Use of topical antimicrobials and antibiotics 70
- **30** Application of lotions, creams, emollients and ointments 74
- **31** Advanced technologies 76

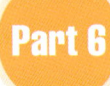

Part 6 Complexities of wound care 79

- **32** Pressure redistribution equipment 80
- **33** Pressure ulcer classification and prevention 82
- **34** Pressure ulcers 86
- **35** Venous leg ulcers 88
- **36** Lymphoedema 90
- **37** Compression therapy 92
- **38** Arterial ulcers 94
- **39** Assessing for arterial disease: ankle–brachial pressure index and toe–brachial pressure index 96
- **40** Interpreting ABPIs 100
- **41** Diabetic foot ulcers 102
- **42** Moisture lesions 106
- **43** Surgical wounds 108
- **44** Traumatic wounds 112
- **45** Burns and scalds 114
- **46** Atypical wounds 116
- **47** Wounds in different populations 118
- **48** Malignant wounds and palliative wound care 120

Glossary 124
References and further reading 126
Index 128

Preface to the second edition

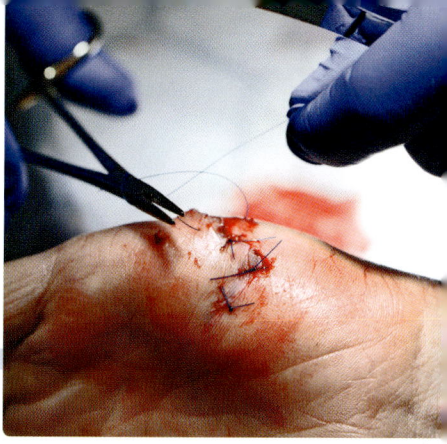

This second edition of *Wound Care at a Glance* has been revised and reviewed in light of the on-going developments in wound care practice. In preparing this new edition, we have listened to readers' feedback, which has encouraged us to provide updates to the chapters in order to reflect changes and advances in the field, and we have added an extended reference list so as to support practice with an evidence base. As wound care management develops, it is also a requirement that nurses and other health care practitioners update their knowledge base as they respond to the needs of the people they offer care and support to. The field of wound care is a dynamic and ever-changing field; keeping up-to-date, and ensuring that care provision is safe, effective and patient centred, are key requirements of any practicing nurse (Nursing and Midwifery Council, 2018).

In order to provide wound care to people across the lifespan, from all socioeconomic backgrounds and in all care specialities and communities, the nurse has to be confident and competent. There is need to understand the anatomy and physiology of the skin, as well as to adopt a holistic and patient-centred approach. This edition again emphasises that wound care has to incorporate patient care. This must involve and engage patients and their families with regards to decisions about their health and care, as this has the potential to enhance individual well-being and care outcomes. When the nurse understands the patient's experiences of the services provided, this can help identify areas of waste and inefficiency, as well how to make improvements to the overall patient experience. When there is a breakdown in skin integrity, this is likely to have a negative impact on the person's health and well-being, as well as the individual's family and society. There will also be implications for the wider health and care economy.

There are often a wide range of professional challenges associated with wound care – from the technological aspects of care to the ethical and sociological questions that should be and are always present when a nurse makes clinical decisions. The provision of high-quality, safe and effective, patient-centred wound care is complex, and success will depend on effective integration of scientific breakthroughs and wound care practices. The provision of wound care and the promotion of wound healing is very much interdisciplinary in nature.

This second edition of *Wound Care at a Glance* retains its easy-to-access approach. This book stays true to the underlying philosophy of the 'At a Glance' series by providing the reader with full-colour illustrations and bite-size information that is easy to digest, as the authors are fully aware that keeping up-to-date with the latest developments in the science of wound care can often be overpowering.

The book has six parts, starting with the history of wound care, the anatomy and physiology, and the normal and abnormal healing processes. The section in the book on wound management in practice emphasises the need for a holistic assessment of skin and describes the various classifications of wounds; in this section, there are chapters dedicated to the ethical and legal aspects of wound care, as well as treatment options and pain management strategies. Dressing selection is a multifaceted process, and the nurse is required to bring together knowledge and understanding of the person as well as the many dressings that are available. Dressing selection and the factors that are required to be taken into consideration when choosing an appropriate wound care product are discussed. There is an emphasis throughout on ensuring that the person's individual needs are addressed. The concluding section of the text takes into account wound care complexities and considers a range of circumstances that the nurse may face.

We were delighted to have been asked to prepare a second edition and have been enthused by the feedback. We are indebted to Wyn Glencross, co-editor of the first edition. Our wish is that this text helps you enhance your practice, knowledge, skills and understanding of wound care.

References

Nursing and Midwifery Council (2018). The Code. Professional standards of practice and behaviour for nurses, midwives and nursing associates. https://www.nmc.org.uk/globalassets/sitedocuments/nmc-publications/nmc-code.pdf. Last accessed September 2019.

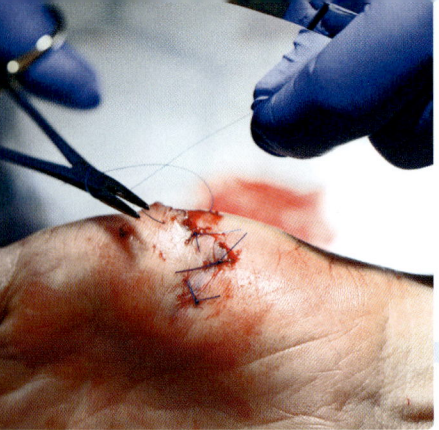

Acknowledgements

Ian would like to thank his partner Jussi Lahtinen for his continued support and Mrs Frances Cohen for her ongoing assistance. Melanie would like to thank Ian for asking her to contribute to the second edition, and her husband James and children Jacob and Amber for their continued support.

We would like to acknowledge the contribution made by Wyn Glencross to the first edition.

How to use your textbook

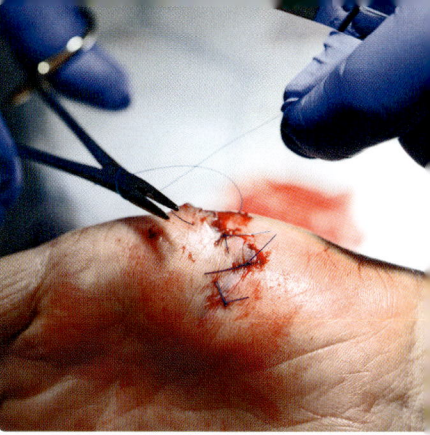

Features contained within your textbook

Each topic is presented in a double-page spread with clear, easy-to-follow diagrams supported by succinct explanatory text.

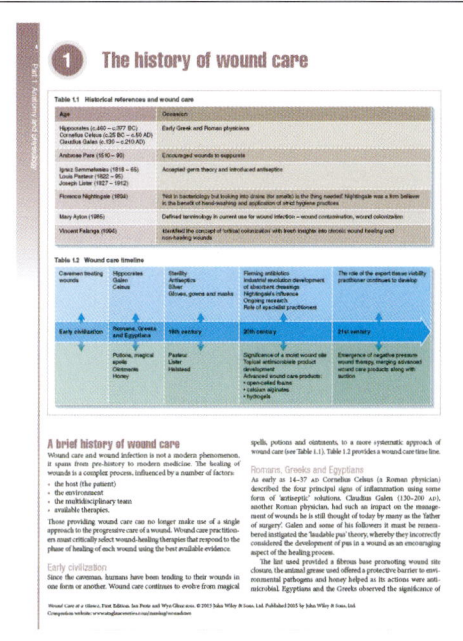

The website icon indicates that you can find accompanying resources on the book's companion website.

Your textbook is full of **photographs, illustrations and tables.**

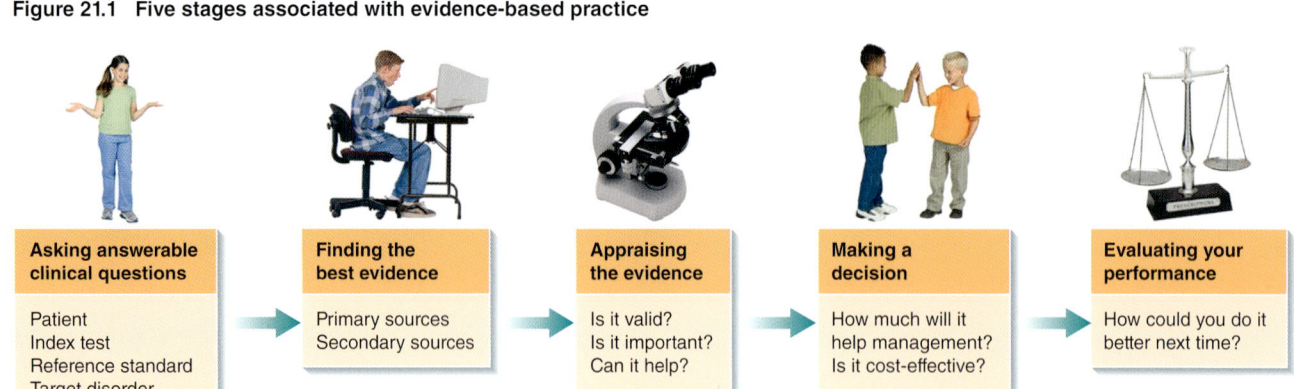

Figure 21.1 Five stages associated with evidence-based practice

Asking answerable clinical questions
Patient
Index test
Reference standard
Target disorder

Finding the best evidence
Primary sources
Secondary sources

Appraising the evidence
Is it valid?
Is it important?
Can it help?

Making a decision
How much will it help management?
Is it cost-effective?

Evaluating your performance
How could you do it better next time?

Source: Thompson and Van den Bruel 2011, figure on p. x of Introduction. Reproduced with permission of Wiley & Sons, Ltd.

Table 21.1 Hierarchy of evidence

Level	Description of evidence	Strength
I	Systematic review or meta-analysis of all relevant randomized controlled trials (RCTs), or evidence-based clinical practice guidelines based on systematic reviews of RCTs	Strongest
II	Evidence from at least one well-designed RCT	
III	Evidence from well-designed controlled trials without randomization	
IV	Evidence from well-designed case-control and cohort studies	
V	Systematic reviews of descriptive and qualitative studies	
VI	A single descriptive or qualitative study	
VII	The opinion of authorities and/or reports of expert committees	Weakest

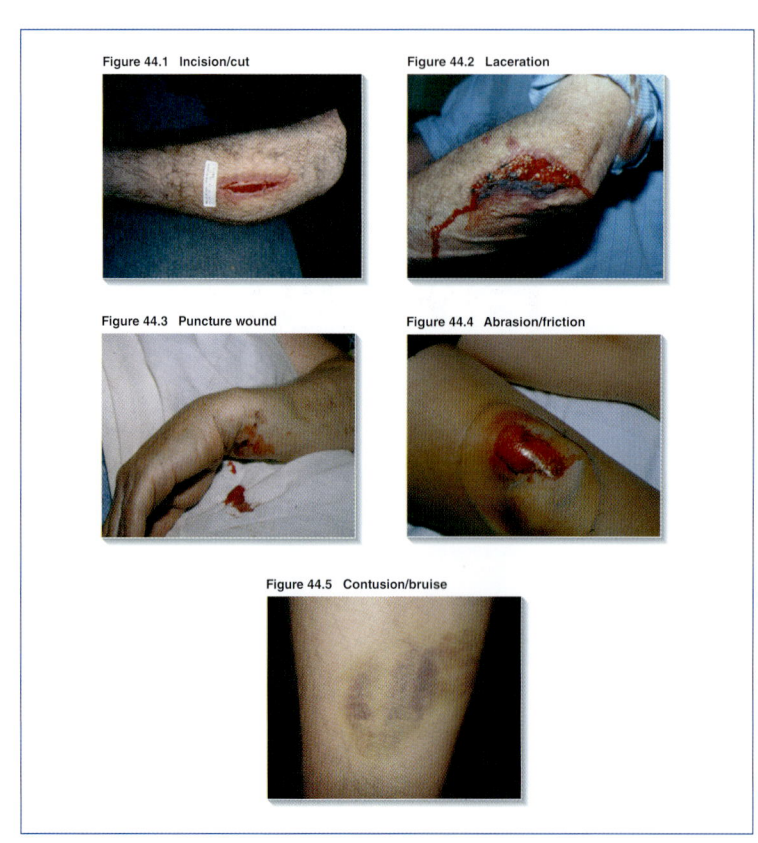

Figure 44.1 Incision/cut
Figure 44.2 Laceration
Figure 44.3 Puncture wound
Figure 44.4 Abrasion/friction
Figure 44.5 Contusion/bruise

About the companion website

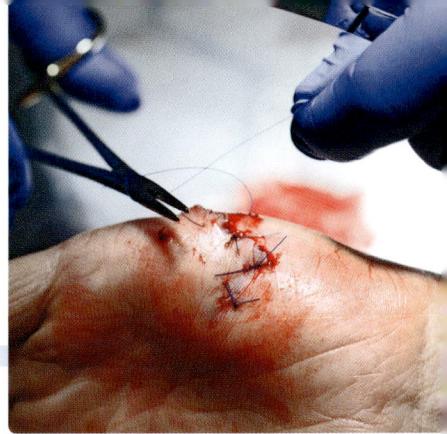

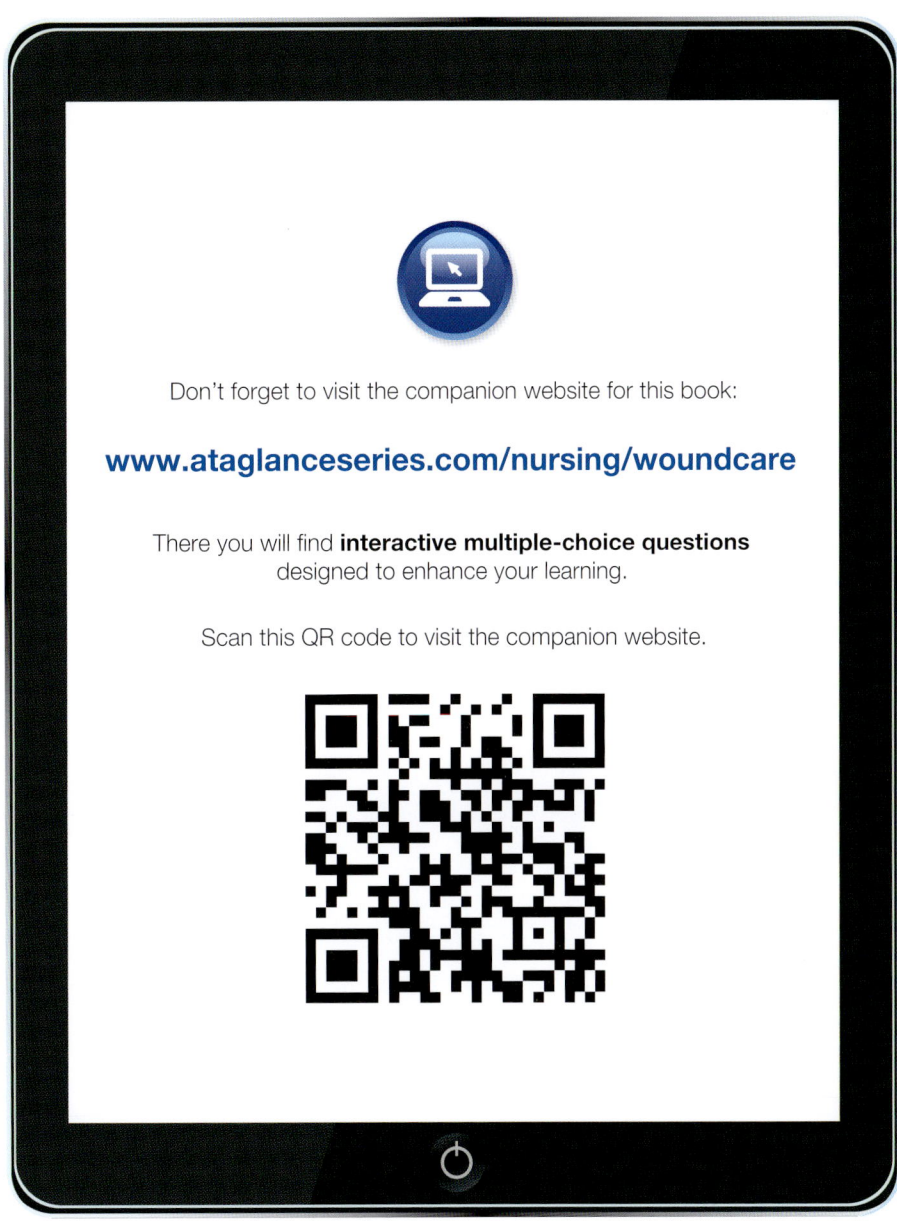

Don't forget to visit the companion website for this book:

www.ataglanceseries.com/nursing/woundcare

There you will find **interactive multiple-choice questions** designed to enhance your learning.

Scan this QR code to visit the companion website.

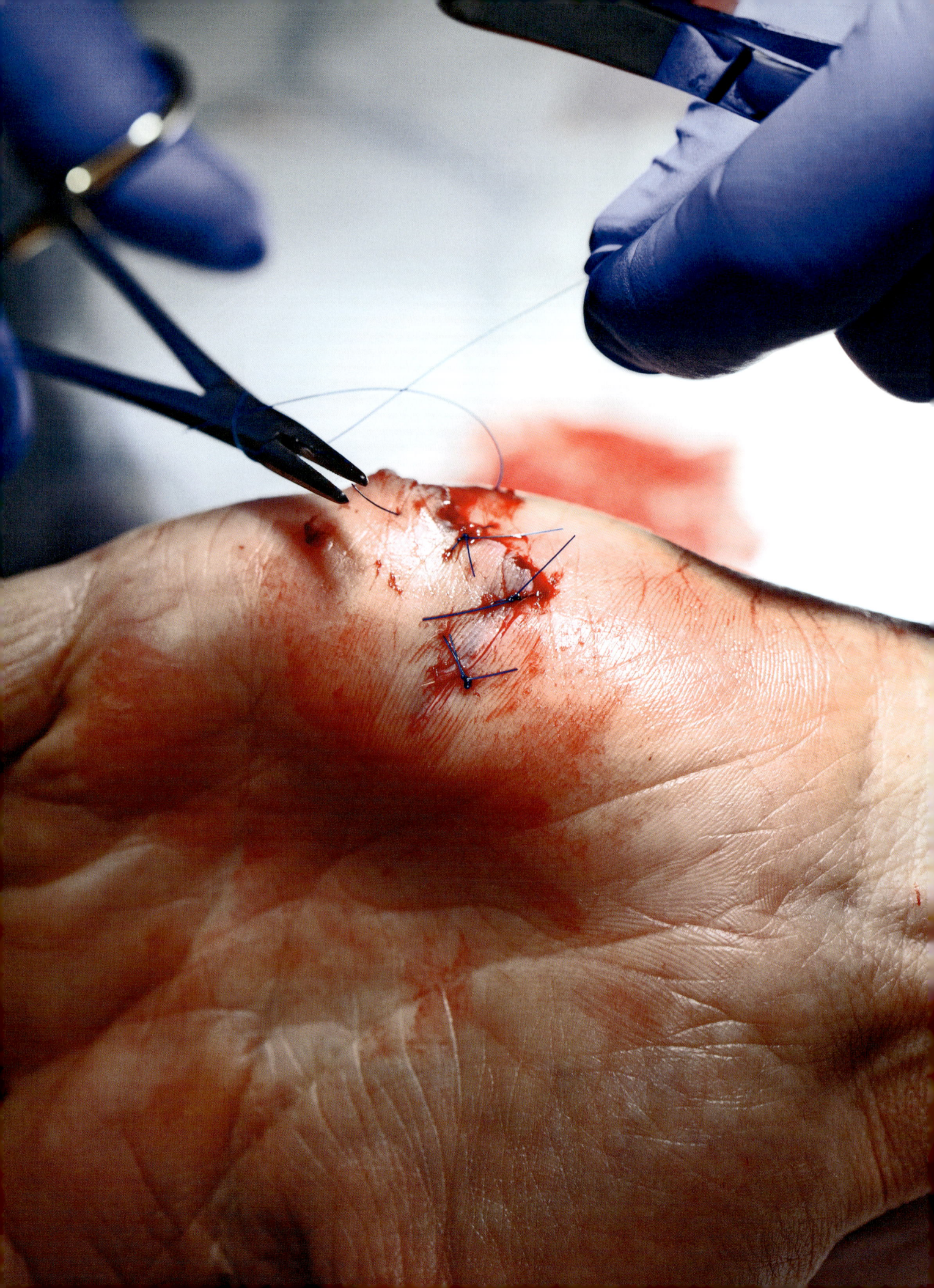

Anatomy and physiology

Chapters

1. The history of wound care 2
2. Anatomy and physiology of the skin 4
3. Psychological and social aspects of the skin 6
4. Body image 8
5. The skin and ageing 12

 Visit the companion website at **www.ataglanceseries.com/nursing/woundcare** to test yourself on these topics.

1 The history of wound care

Table 1.1 Historical references and wound care.

Age	Occasion
Hippocrates (c. 460–c. 377 BC) Cornelius Celsus (c. 25 BC–c. 50 AD) Claudius Galen (c. 130–c. 210 AD)	Early Greek and Roman physicians Wine or vinegar was used to cleanse wounds, and the follow-up treatment included the application of honey, oil and wine
Ambrose Pare (1510–1590)	Encouraged wounds to suppurate
Ignaz Semmelweiss (1818–1865) Louis Pasteur (1822–1895) Joseph Lister (1827–1912)	Accepted the germ theory and the introduction of antiseptics
Florence Nightingale (1894)	'Not in bacteriology, but looking into drains (for smells) is the thing needed'. Nightingale was a firm believer in the benefits of sanitation, hand-washing and application of strict hygiene practices
George D. Winter (1962)	Discovered the importance of moist wound-healing in experimental animals
Mary Ayton (1985)	Defined the terminology that is currently used for wound infection – wound contamination and wound colonisation
Vincent Falanga (1994)	Identified the concept of 'critical colonisation' with fresh insights into chronic wound-healing and non-healing wounds

Table 1.2 Wound care timeline.

Cave dwellers treating wounds	Hippocrates Galen Celsus	Sterility Antiseptics Silver Gloves, gowns and masks	Fleming antibiotics Industrial Revolution Development of absorbent dressings Nightingale's influence Ongoing research Role of specialist practitioners	The role of the expert tissue viability practitioner continues to grow
Early civilisation	**Romans, Greeks and Egyptians**	**19th century**	**20th century**	**21st century**
	Potions, magical spells Ointments Honey	Pasteur Lister Halstead	Significance of a moist wound site Topical antimicrobials product development Advanced wound care products: • Open-celled foams • Calcium alginates • Hydrogels	Emergence of negative pressure wound therapy; merging advanced wound care products along with suction

Wound Care at a Glance, Second Edition. Ian Peate and Melanie Stephens.
© 2020 John Wiley & Sons Ltd. Published 2020 by John Wiley & Sons Ltd.
Companion website: http://www.ataglanceseries.com/nursing/woundcare/

A brief history of wound care

Wound care and infection is not a modern phenomenon; it spans from pre-history to modern medicine. The healing of wounds is a complex process, influenced by a number of factors:

- The host (the patient)
- The environment
- The multidisciplinary team
- Available therapies.

Those providing wound care can no longer stick to a single approach in the progressive care of a wound. Wound care practitioners must critically select such wound-healing therapies that can respond to the healing phase of any wound using the best available evidence. For thousands of years, dressing materials have been continually developing so as to provide protection, absorption and act as a base for wound bed preparation. Over the last 30 years, the advances in would care have been more prolific as compared to the previous 2000 years.

Early civilisation

Since the era of cave dwellers, humans have been tending to their wounds in one form or another. Wound care continues to evolve from casting magical spells and applying potions and ointments to a more systematic approach (see Table 1.1). See Table 1.2 for the wound care timeline.

Romans, greeks and egyptians

As early as 14–37 AD, Cornelius Celsus (a Roman physician) described the four principal signs of inflammation using some form of 'antiseptic' solutions. Claudius Galen (130–200 AD), another Roman physician, had such expertise on the management of healing wounds that he is still considered the 'father of surgery' by many. Galen and some of his followers must be remembered for instigating the 'laudable pus' theory, whereby they incorrectly considered the development of pus in a wound as an encouraging aspect of the healing process.

The lint provided a fibrous base promoting the covering of a wound site, the animal grease offered a protective barrier to the environmental pathogens, and the honey helped with its antimicrobial actions. The Egyptians and Greeks observed the significance of covering a wound. The Greeks were the first to identify the difference between acute and chronic wounds, correspondingly calling them 'fresh' and 'non-healing'. Around 120–201 AD, a Greek surgeon, who served the Roman gladiators, made a number of contributions to wound care by successfully covering a moist wound site and recognising its importance.

After the fall of the Roman Empire, many of these advances were lost. In the Middle Ages in Europe, there was a regression in the field of wound care, returning to the use of potions and charms.

The use of honey as a wound care treatment has recently seen a revival. Ancient Egyptians used honey as a wound treatment as early as 3000 BC, and its traces have been found in Egyptian tombs. Honey is said to have been an essential part of the 'Three Healing Gestures' used by the Egyptians.

19th century

Pasteur's theories were associated with the impact of microbes on diseases, and the use of phenol by Lister introduced the modern 'germ theory' when he demonstrated the beneficial effects of carbolic acid (phenol) in the dressings of infected wounds at the turn of the century. Halstead introduced the wearing of gloves, gowns and masks, and silver was revived as an antiseptic used in dressings, enhancing the healing of wounds.

All of these events make the 19th century a significant and eventful era with regard to advances within the field of sterility and sterile surgical procedures. Skin cleaning, the use of antiseptics and debridement became common practices thereafter.

20th century

The 20th century brought some key advances, when there was a resurgence and rediscovery of the significance of a moist wound site with the invention and development of polymer synthetics used for wound dressings.

Fleming's discovery and the subsequent development of antibiotics provided us with potent antimicrobial therapies with high specificity, transforming clinical therapy and marking the decline of a number of former remedies. Yet, the emergence of antibiotic-resistant strains of pathogens, alongside the delayed discovery of newer antibiotics, led to a need for the discovery and development of alternative treatments.

Topical antimicrobials in the current wound care practice include iodine- and silver-containing products. In the past, acetic acid, chlorhexidine, hydrogen peroxide, sodium hypochlorite, potassium permanganate and proflavine have been used. Some of these are making a comeback, and other options are being investigated and considered.

During the 1800s in the UK, natural products were being refined, leading to the development of absorbent natural products for dressings, including spun and woven cotton. During the First World War, absorbent dressings were being manufactured. Tulle gras, a paraffin gauze dressing, was developed by Lumière. Plastics were being added to cotton in the 1950s creating composite dressings, such as plasters. Throughout this timeframe, the key aim was to dry out the wound, focusing upon protection and absorption, reducing the trauma of dressing changes. There is much evidence to suggest that keeping wounds moist is more effective to letting them dry out.

Advanced wound care products were being designed in the 1970s taking advantage of this concept; nurses were using these products to successfully treat chronic wounds. Much research was undertaken in the late 1970s and 1980s.

In early 1980s, hydrocolloid, the second advanced dressing, was developed. Hydrocolloid wafers were established as first-line treatment for pressure ulcers, leading to the development of more absorbent dressings, for example, foams and alginates.

The late 1980s witnessed the introduction of other advanced wound care products:

- Open-celled foams
- Calcium alginates
- Hydrogels.

Nurses began to take the lead with wound care or tissue viability, managing and organizing outpatient wound clinics, influencing and enhancing patient care.

Product diversification and growth continued throughout the 1990s. Sustained-release antimicrobial dressings were beginning to emerge and growth factor impregnated hydrogel as well as living skin equivalents.

21st century

Product modification continued throughout the 2000s, and this will continue with the emergence of negative pressure wound therapy and merging advanced wound care products along with suction.

The future

The field of medicine is constantly evolving with advancements in wound care techniques. A number of new laboratory tools have provided us with the ability to gather an incredible amount of scientific data related to the biological events associated with healing. Much more needs to be accomplished in this field, as pieces of the jigsaw, fitting together in a way that is important for the patient, are still missing. The future is unknown, but the people requiring wound care will still need a kind of treatment that is kind and compassionate.

Anatomy and physiology of the skin

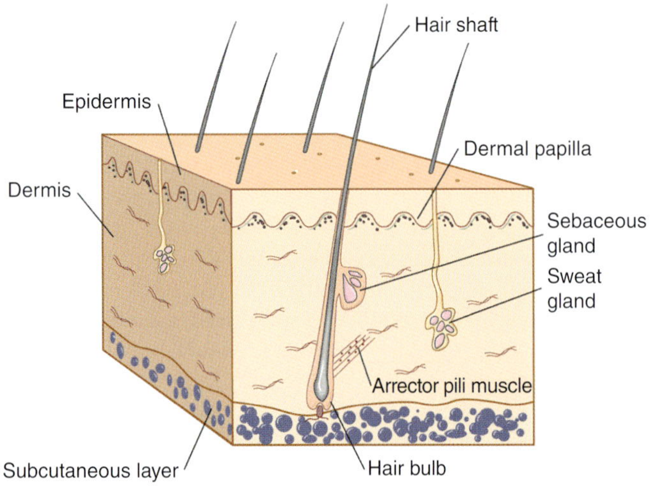

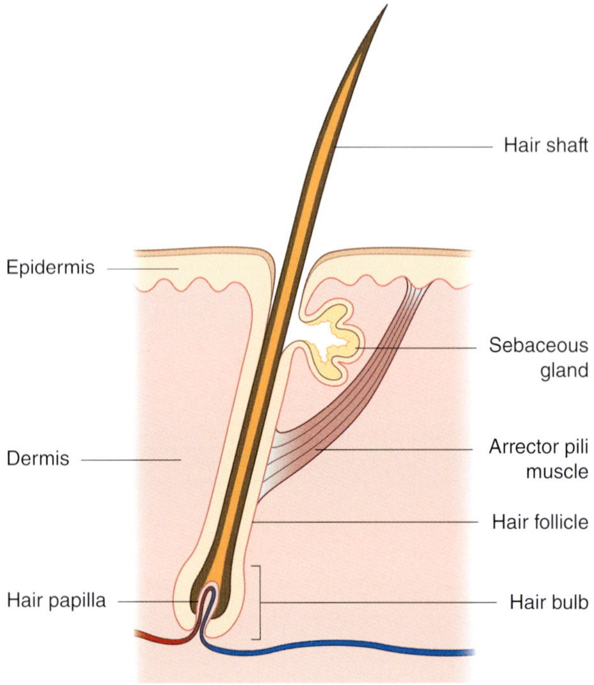

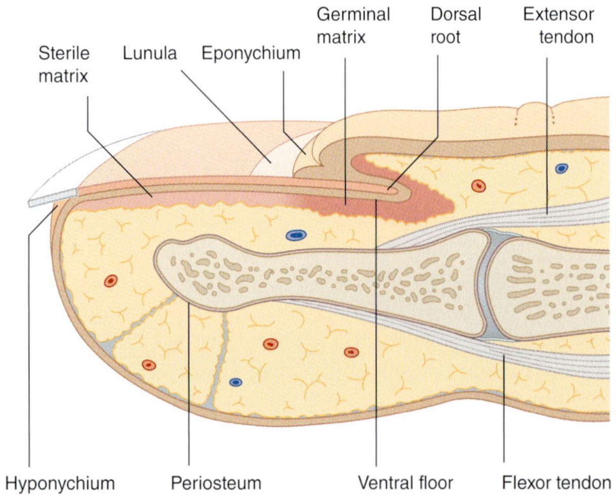

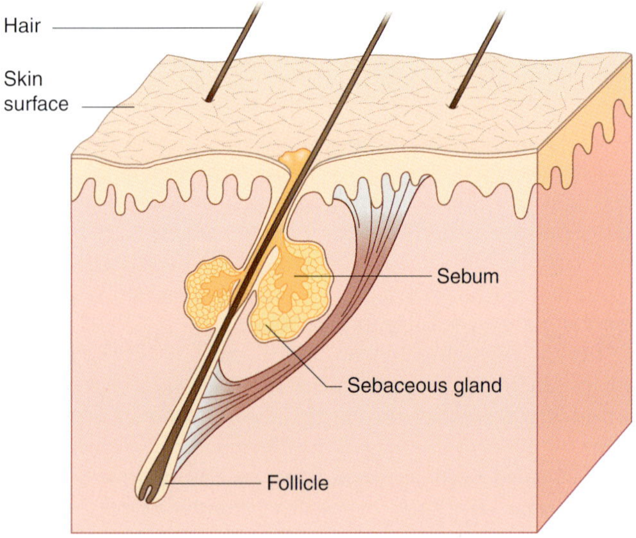

The skin is the largest organ of the body, consisting of accessory organs such as glands, hair and nails (the appendages). It is a multifunctional organ:

- It protects against biological invasion, physical damage and ultraviolet radiation.
- Nerve endings provide sensation.
- It provides thermoregulation through sweating and the regulation of blood flow.
- It synthesises Vitamin D.
- Sweat excretes salts and small amounts of waste.
- Aesthetics and communication.

The skin has three layers: the epidermis (Figure 2.1), the dermis and the hypodermis. Skin health has a great impact on the overall health of the individual, and it is of profound psychological importance.

Epidermis

This predominantly consists of stratified epithelium; the outer layer continually sheds dead cells and is slightly acidic with pH 4.5–6. The basal layer constantly forms new cells, gradually moving towards the surface and flattening during this process, prior to being shed from the skin surface; this can take between 28 and 35 days. Depending on their location, these cells are normally four or five layers thick, and most layers are present on the palms and the soles.

Layers of the epidermis

The epidermis is divided into five layers: stratum corneum, stratum lucidum, stratum granulosum, stratum spinosum and stratum basale.

- *Stratum corneum*: Tough, waterproof uppermost layer, consists of fibrous dead cells, assists with the maintenance of pH and temperature and has a protective role to play. The continual replacement of the millions of worn out cells contributes to the skin's ability to repair itself.
- *Stratum lucidum*: Not always present in some areas of the body and appears where skin is thinner. Provides extra protection in those areas exposed to wear and tear.
- *Stratum granulosum*: In this layer, keratinocytes lose their nuclei and start to flatten and die; keratinisation takes place here. The stratum granulosum helps reduce loss of water from the epidermis.
- *Stratum spinosum*: Contains living cells with spiny processes called *desmosomes*. The stratum spinosum is 8–10 cells thick.
- *Stratum basale*: Also known as the basement membrane, this is the lowest layer. This layer is one cell thick, forming a definitive border between the dermis and the epidermis. Cells at this level continually divide and develop, providing ongoing rejuvenation of the skin. Melanocytes are produced here.

Dermis

The key purpose of the dermis is to support and provide nutrition to the epidermis.

The key component of the dermis is proteinous connective tissue made up of the arc-shaped elastic fibres and undulated and practically inelastic collagen fibres (elastin). Other elements include fibroblasts, mast cells, other tissue cells, multiple blood and lymph vessels, nerve endings, hot and cold receptors and tactile sensory organs.

The dermis contains blood capillaries, sensory nerve endings, lymphatic vessels, sweat glands, sebaceous glands and hair follicles.

The flexible irregular connective tissue made from woven collagen and elastin fibres abound with blood vessels, nerve fibres and lymphatic vessels. Ridges formed from these bundles of collagen run downward, forward and horizontally around the body and are called *cleavage lines*; they are genetically determined and are unique for each person.

Hypodermis

The superficial facia provides anchorage to the skin whilst allowing some capacity for it to move. It offers support to the dermis and is made up primarily of adipose tissue, connective tissue and blood vessels. The fat stored within the hypodermis offers protection to the internal structures, insulating against cold.

Appendages

Hair

Made up of keratin, at the lower end is a bulb or root enclosed in a follicle that produces the hair. The root is indented by a hair papilla, connective tissue and blood vessels. The hair follicle is an epithelium-lined sheath, the arrector pilli (smooth muscle) extends through the dermis, attached to the base of the follicle, and the hair stands on the end when the muscle contracts (Figure 2.2).

There are no hair on the palms of the hands, soles of the feet, nails, parts of the external genitals, lips and nipples. Protection of the skin by hair is constrained; however, its role is to protect the scalp specifically from ultraviolet rays, heat loss and injury. The eyebrows and the eyelashes offer protection from foreign bodies entering the eye.

Nails

The nails are a specialised type of keratin, situated over the distal surfaces of fingers and toes. The nail plate is surrounded on three ends by cuticles (see Figure 2.3).

The function of nails is to assist with the development of fine motor skills, such as grasping, scratching and manipulation. The nails provide protection against trauma to the fingers and toes.

Sebaceous glands

These are located on all parts of the skin except palms and soles; they are more prominent on the scalp, face, upper torso and genitalia, producing sebum, made up of keratin, fat and cellulose debris. Sebum forms a moist, oily acidic film that has antibacterial and antifungal properties (Figure 2.4).

Blood vessels

The blood vessels include arterioles, capillary networks and venules. Blood vessels in the skin are responsible for the transportation and distribution of oxygen, nutrients and hormones, as well as for the removal of waste products.

Nerve fibres

Both the sensory and motor nerves are present within the dermis. The sensory nerve endings are sensitive to touch, or initiate signals producing sensations of warmth, coolness, pain, pressure, vibration, tickling and itching.

Lymphatic vessels

The lymphatic system matches the supply and function of blood vessels.

3 Psychological and social aspects of the skin

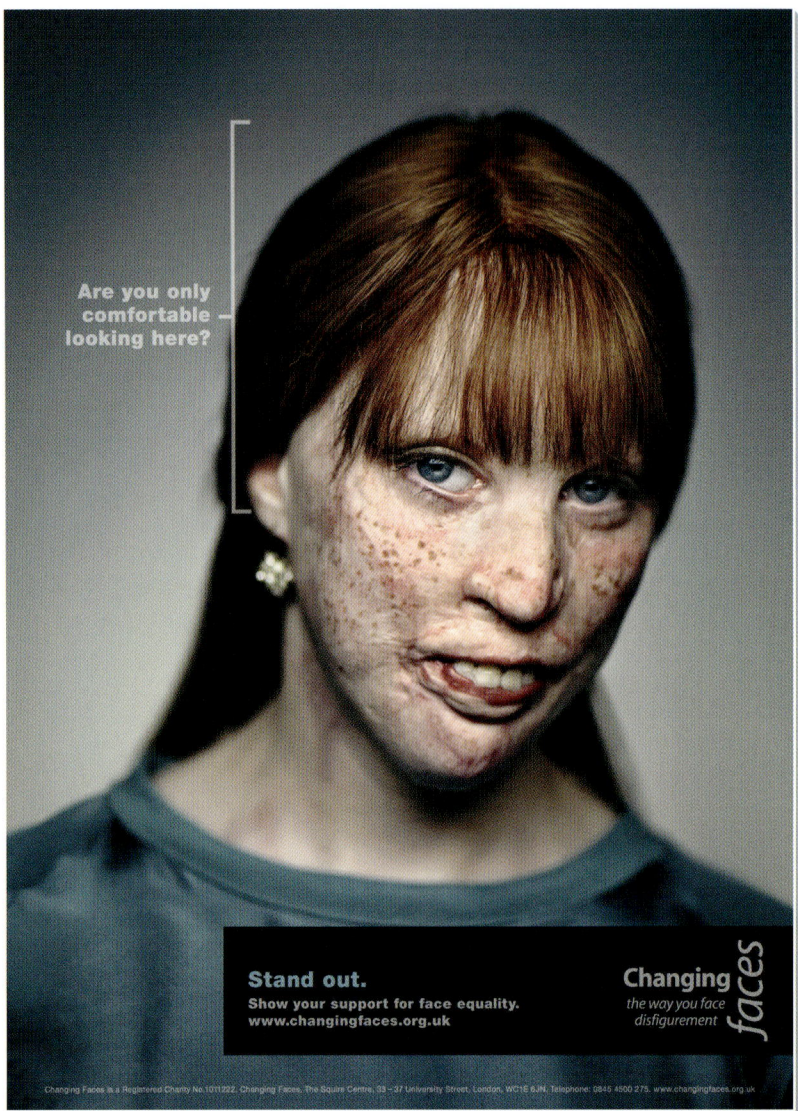

Figure 3.1 Changing Faces campaign poster.

Source: Changing Faces 2008.

Case study: Anil

As a result of a road traffic accident when a child, Anil sustained a significant disfiguring scar on his left cheek; the scar had faded over time. When he was younger, Anil was very uncomfortable when having his picture taken or when he saw himself in the mirror; if somebody stared at him, he felt he was being mocked. Recently, as an adult, Anil was hospitalised with shortness of breath. During the ward round where the medical team was discussing Anil's condition, he was very self-conscious and felt he was being criticised and judged. Because of this, Anil became less responsive and less willing to provide any information that could have contributed to his care. As a child, Anil was social, interactive and playful until he was involved in the accident at the age of 5 years. Anil's body image as an adult reflected his early response to trauma and disfigurement.

The skin – psychological and social aspects

The physical presence of the skin as the largest organ of the body is significant in relation to the psychological and social perspectives of a person. The skin has psychological and social components; its appearance can lead to discrimination and also has the ability to reveal a person's state of health and well-being. The relationship between the skin, the mind and the individual has been the subject of study for several years. When practitioners understand this complex relationship, they are then be able to offer assistance with regard to the various coping mechanisms that can be used by people to help them live with wounds – healed or healing. Self-harm, its manifestations and its treatment are addressed in Part 6.

Stress and anxiety

Psychological stress and physiological stress (for whatever reason) can change the wound-healing process. Psychological stress can have a significant clinical impact on wound repair.

Wound-healing processes can be directly impacted by the physiological stress response, whereas psychological stress can impact indirectly resulting in a modification of the repair process; this may occur by the promotion of health-damaging behaviours being adopted by the person.

Wound-healing is an important aspect concerned with the recovery from injury and surgical interventions. If healing is negatively impacted, it can increase the risk of:

- Developing wound infections
- Developing other complications
- Increasing the duration of hospital stay
- Increasing patient discomfort
- Delaying the patient's ability to perform the activities of living and returning to independence.

A significant number of people suffer some form of psychological distress after sustaining a wound or any damage to skin integrity. The person may experience the impact of an altered body image, and this can lead the person feeling devalued by society as well as by those close to them.

A wound in the process of healing or having healed resulting in scar formation can lead to the person believing that they are a social leper and feeling that others do not want to mix or be associated with them. The person's quality of life can be adversely affected.

Anxiety

Anxiety can be associated with a number of things, for example:

- Uncertainty
- Admission to hospital
- Fear of pain
- Fear of death
- Fear of the unknown.

While some degree of anxiety may be beneficial, excessive and prolonged anxiety can lead to psychological and physiological dysfunction. Anxiety and depression tools can be used to help assess and identify the levels of stress experienced. Assessment results can help the practitioner and patient to formulate a plan that will assist in relieving the anxiety and stress being experienced.

Practitioners should consider assessing and reassessing the patient's psychological state as part of the overall plan of care. It is essential to make a baseline observation and then compare consecutive observations with the baseline.

Emotional impact

The physical discomfort and the morbidity often caused by wounds also have an emotional effect on the person, the people delivering care, family members, friends and onlookers. Wounds are often viewed negatively, and patients may feel unattractive, vulnerable, contagious, imperfect and in some instances repulsive. Wounds can be seen as appalling, scary, time-consuming, costly, smelly, dirty, disfiguring, uncomfortable and unpleasant; people can feel humiliated, embarrassed, guilty and shamed because of wounds. All of this can lead to extreme self-consciousness and social isolation.

Management

A multidisciplinary approach is required. A competent psychological assessment and input assures the patients that they are valued, and this can lead to positive health care outcomes. Management strategies should incorporate such interventions that minimise patient distress, including the provision of social support and the development of coping skills. A psychosomatic approach should combine psychological therapy as well as physical therapy that considers the person holistically. The aim should be to eliminate pain if present and consider pharmacological interventions and the physical and psychological components; this must be tailored to each patient's needs. Failing to address issues such as pain can make depression worse and impact further on a person's self esteem.

Cognitive behavioural therapy

The psychological intervention that has the greatest evidence for success is cognitive behavioural therapy (CBT), which includes stress management, problem-solving, meditation, relaxation and goal-setting. In CBT, therapists help patients:

- With their communication skills
- Provide a sense of control
- Cope with the fear of pain and rejection.

This is done through learning positive coping strategies and will go some way to improving the person's mood.

CBT, a talking therapy, focuses on the present and aims to change thoughts and behaviours in order to improve mental health and well-being. The central principle of CBT is that it can change thought and behavioural patterns, having a significant impact on a person's emotions; this approach can help people identify and analyse any counter-productive thoughts and behaviours they may have. A skilled and trained therapist working with the patient can help to ease feelings of anxiety or depression. CBT is recommended by the National Institute for Health and Care Excellence, which has provided guidelines for its use relating to disorders, such as anxiety.

Referral

An appropriate referral may need to be made to other agencies, such as a counsellor, psychotherapist or to external agencies within the third sector, such as the charitable organisation, Changing Faces, http://www.changingfaces.org.uk/ (Figure 3.1).

4 Body image

Figure 4.1 The impact of a wound on a person's self-esteem and body image.

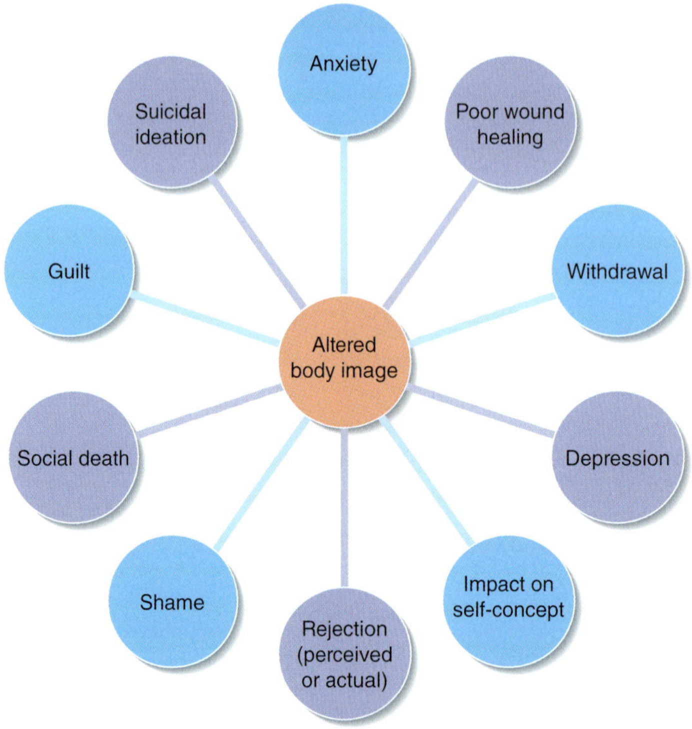

Altered body image:
- Anxiety
- Poor wound healing
- Withdrawal
- Depression
- Impact on self-concept
- Rejection (perceived or actual)
- Shame
- Social death
- Guilt
- Suicidal ideation

Table 4.1 Examples of communication strategies for addressing body image concerns (source: Adapted from Fingerert 2014).

	Body image challenge	Typical responses	Preferred responses	
			Exploratory phrases	**Empathic phrases**
1.	'I can't bear to look in the mirror or show my body to my wife since I had my mastectomy'.	You look smashing! Don't worry, the swelling will continue to go down and, in a couple of weeks, things will look even better.	What is it that you see when you look in the mirror? Have you discussed your worries with your wife?	This must be a big change for you, as you used to be more comfortable with your body.
2.	'I rarely leave the house any more since my surgery. I don't like it when people stare at me or talk about my appearance or my garbled speech. I worry about what others think of me, particularly my grandchildren'.	You need to get out more, and then you will feel much better. Your family still needs you and they love you just the way you are.	What do you think your grandchildren think of you now? Do you think your friends and family miss seeing you?	It is obvious that you love your grandchildren a lot. It must be difficult for you to not spend time with them as you used to do.

Wound Care at a Glance, Second Edition. Ian Peate and Melanie Stephens.
© 2020 John Wiley & Sons Ltd. Published 2020 by John Wiley & Sons Ltd.
Companion website: http://www.ataglanceseries.com/nursing/woundcare/

Case study: Carry Anne

A malignant fungating breast wound is an infiltration of a cancer or metastasis into the skin and the afferent blood and lymph vessels in the breast. Unless the malignant cells are brought under control, through treatment with chemotherapy, radiotherapy or hormone therapy, the fungation may spread outwards by local extension causing damage through a combination of loss of vascularity, proliferative growth and ulceration. Damage is also caused to the patient's psychological well-being.

Carry Anne, 71 years old, was admitted to the surgical ward via the emergency department with an initial diagnosis of malignant fungating breast wound. Carry Anne had delayed seeking help and tried to hide the reality of the cancer. The wound she said has had a huge impact causing her shame. Carry Anne told the nurse that she has given up, feels dirty and no longer feels like a woman. Initially Carry Anne tried to manage the wound herself, but the symptoms had caused revulsion, and this had a significant impact on her psychological well-being. She was embarrassed by the symptoms, and this had taken its toll on her social life. Carry Anne told the nurse about failing to seek medical help, as she was scared this could be cancer.

The visibility of the wound and the odour caused Carry Anne immense distress and changed her relationships with family and friends. She had stopped inviting people to her home, was embarrassed, and had not gone out in over 8 months; she was socially isolated. Carry Anne said she wanted to die.

A wound care clinical nurse specialist undertook an assessment of Carry Anne's physical and psychological needs; there was excessive exudate and leakage, and the odour emanating from the wound was unpleasant. Carry Anne was in pain and the wound site was bleeding. She was constantly itching or wanting to itch. It was evident that Carry Anne was severely depressed, as she had no interest in the care that was being planned or offered. Malignant fungating wounds cause enormous distress and they are associated with significant morbidity. The life expectancy for a person living with such a wound is very short.

The overall aim of the care plan was to make Carry Anne more comfortable, to be less distressed and to reduce the experience of stigma and social isolation as the wound-related symptoms are managed. Malignant wounds do not heal, and in Carry Anne's case she was cared for using palliative methods to control both wound-related symptoms and to manage her pain. Carry Anne died 6 days after admission to the ward.

Body image

In contemporary Western societies, appearances in general and specifically the body image have become central and important concepts. The strong emphasis on the appearance and a beautiful body is very much evident when media images are examined, shop windows are looked at, magazines flicked through and websites visited. The amount of money spent in the pursuit of beauty through dieting, aesthetic surgical procedures and everyday grooming practices reinforces the emphasis placed on the appearance and its esteem.

The body image is associated with the mental representation or perception that we create of what we think we look like; it can or may not bear a close relation to how others really see us; it may be very different from a person's actual physical appearance. Body image is subjected to many different kinds of distortions that can come from internal factors, such as our emotions, moods, our early experiences, the attitudes of our parents and more. However, it has a strong influence on behaviour. Infatuation with and distortions of body image are widespread among those people (as well as onlookers) who have a wound or have a scar that has formed as a result of a wound.

All those with wounds will experience some form of altered body image, and this in turn can have an effect on a person's sense of self-esteem. A person's social and psychological well-being is in danger of being threatened, and as such his/her quality of life can be impacted in a negative and detrimental way. Those wounds that result in disfigurement are

- Amputation
- Mastectomy
- Burns
- Formation of ostomy.

These wounds can profoundly alter the mental picture a person has of him or her – the body image. This is confounded further, as that person may be anxious about the unknown and its prognosis.

Disfiguring surgery, such as mastectomy or amputation, brings with it a dramatic change in body image; this coupled with the diagnosis of a life-threatening condition such as cancer can leave a person vulnerable. Those who have undergone disfiguring surgery with, for example, the loss of a body part may be experiencing and going through the grieving process and having to deal with a number of mixed emotions, such as:

- Loss
- Anxiety
- Withdrawal of social relationships
- Depression
- Suicidal ideation.

Natural changes to body image, for example, the changes that are associated with puberty and ageing, are generally the expected changes, but any development from a wound may not be. Altered body image happens when unnatural or unexpected changes in a person's self-concept occur, for example, a wound. Wounds can bring unexpected challenges and are themselves capable of changing the course of a person's life.

The circumstances, the visibility and the severity under which the injury occurred can have a significant effect on a person's acceptance of the wound associated with his or her altered body image (Figure 4.1). Some people have developed coping mechanisms that enable them to think that the wound does not belong to them (objectification).

Management

The response that a person makes to the presence of a wound (patient, healthcare provider or stranger) is unpredictable. Those wounds that are present on the face, hands and neck are often the most difficult to conceal from the viewpoints of others as well as the person himself/herself. Table 4.1 provides the examples of communication strategies for addressing body image concerns.

Assessing the impact of altered body image

Wound assessment should also take into account the assessment of a person's physical and psychological well-being, as both may have a negative impact upon the wound-healing process (see Chapter 3).

Body image can be adversely affected or altered (temporarily or permanently) as a result of a change in a person's physical appearance, such as trauma or the result of surgical intervention. Acute and chronic wounds have the potential to adversely impact on a person's body image and as such their self-esteem.

There are a number of tools and scales that can be used to assess the impact of altered body image on a person. A five-point Likert scale – the Stigma Scale – has been developed that can be used to provide objective assessment as to how a person views their body image. There are different types of stigma, for example:

- Anticipated stigma (perceived stigma)
- Internalised stigma (self-stigma)
- Experienced stigma (discrimination).

When the results of the assessment are analysed, a care pathway can be formulated to help the patients and their families cope with the problems and challenges they may have. The practitioner should aim to establish a person-centred approach that acknowledges any person as a whole. Neglecting the psychological needs of a person may result in a threat to his/her quality of life and the sense of self. The emotional trauma experienced by people with wounds that result in an altered body image due to disfiguration can take many years of adjustment (and in some cases the person may never adjust to the degree of mutilation experienced).

Each change of dressing brings attention to the injured body part; brings with it pain, a reminder of the injury, how this occurred, as well as possible fears about the future. The way a healthcare provider responds to a wound, for example, through acceptance, compassion, disappointment, repulsion, fear or avoidance, can have a detrimental impact on a person's emotional state and his/her self-esteem.

Referral

It may be necessary to make appropriate referrals to other agencies, such as a counsellor or a psychotherapist, or there may be a need to refer to external agencies where services such as skin camouflage can be offered to people in need of help to grow in confidence and independence.

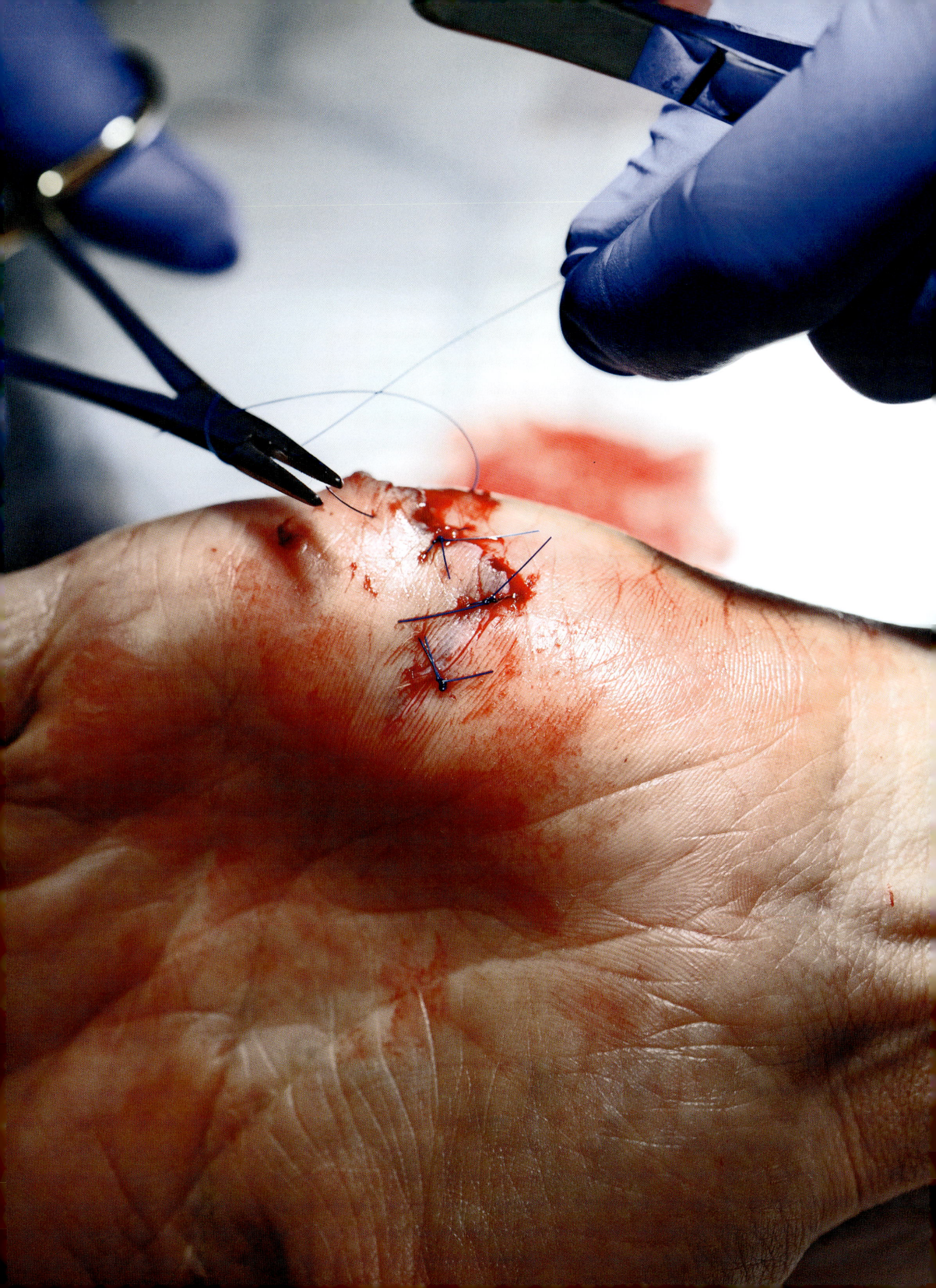

5 The skin and ageing

Table 5.1 Wound-healing and ageing skin.

Effect of ageing on skin	Effect of ageing on healing
Keratinocyte maturation is decreased	Reduction in the ability of the skin to repair Wound contraction decreases
Reduction in the production of melanocytes	When exposed to the sun, reaction of the skin decreases
Merkel cell production is reduced	Sensation is reduced
Dermal/epidermal junction flattens	Likelihood of skin rupture increases resulting in tearing of skin Delivery of nutrients to the epidermis is impaired Microcirculation is diminished Possibility of an increase of shearing and blistering
Reduction in the number of Langerhans cells	Immune response is inhibited or reduced
Diminished sebaceous and sweat gland activity and, therefore, reduction in the production of sebum	Dehydration of the skin Ability to maintain normal acidity is compromised pH of the skin increases Uncharacteristic fissure formation, scaling, cracking and pruritis
The normal barriers of protection lose their effectiveness	Increased vulnerability to harmful irritants Increased vulnerability to developing contact dermatitis Transdermal permeability of water increases
Diminished sensory perception	Difficulty in being able to discern sensations increases
Decreased vascularity	Ability to thermoregulate effectively is impaired Decrease in angiogenesis (capillary growth) Decreased ability to form granulation tissue Impairment in the supply of nutrients to the skin
Dermal atrophy	The skin's protective padding decreases A potential danger of damage and risk to underlying structures

Box 5.1 Skin and ageing.

- There are two types of skin ageing – intrinsic and extrinsic ageing.
- Ageing skin becomes more fragile and loses 20% of its thickness.
- Ageing skin is more fragile and prone to wounding.
- The ageing population is increasing considerably.
- Wound care costs for this group are rising; this, in part, is because the wound care needs of this population are becoming chronic.
- Having an understanding of the impact that ageing can have on skin biology and wound-healing will help nurses tailor care plans so as to address the many physiological manifestations of ageing.

Wound Care at a Glance, Second Edition. Ian Peate and Melanie Stephens.
© 2020 John Wiley & Sons Ltd. Published 2020 by John Wiley & Sons Ltd.
Companion website: http://www.ataglanceseries.com/nursing/woundcare/

Ageing population

There is an ageing population in the UK and other Western countries. The number of people over the age of 65 years is set to rise. Older skin brings with it many challenges related to intrinsic and extrinsic factors.

Skin changes are among the most visible signs of ageing (see Box 5.1). The evidences of increasing age include wrinkles and sagging skin. Another obvious sign of ageing is the whitening or greying of the hair.

At the cellular level

As we age, skin structure and its normal functions go through gradual change. As a result of these structural and functional changes, the ability of tissue to repair becomes impaired and the processes are altered. The contraction ability of a wound and reepithelialisation process slows down, the accumulation of connective tissues diminishes and ultimately the wound's tensile strength decreases. At each layer of the skin, there are specific characteristic changes that occur as we age.

From a histological perspective (at cellular level), the epidermis is thinned along with a loss of the rete ridge and reduction in the amount of Langerhans cells and melanocytes; the remaining melanocytes increase in size. Ageing skin therefore appears thinner, paler and clear (translucent). Large pigmented spots (called age spots, liver spots or lentigos) may appear in sun-exposed areas.

The epidermal cells reduce in size and the dermis becomes thinner, predominantly due to a loss of proteoglycans. From a functional perspective, elasticity and tensile strength are reduced. Risk of damage from injury, irritants and infection increases, and wound-healing occurs at a slower rate. See Table 5.1 for a summary of the changes associated with wound healing and ageing skin.

The epidermis

The epidermis is in a constant state of change with the production of new cells approximately every 28 days. The keratinocytes that are formed in the basement membrane go through chemical and morphological changes as they move through the epidermis, where they eventually shed to make way for a new layer of matured keratinocytes. The number of keratinocytes available to resurface and replace those lost cells decreases as we age. In an older person, the normal maturation rate of the epidermal macrophages – Langerhans cells – is decreased. Apart from this, there is also a decrease in the number of cells that are required to fight off infections.

This decrease in the number of cells acting as first responders in case of infection causes a diminished immune system response. As we age, the normal number of melanocytes that are present in the epidermis decreases; in addition, melanin production within the hair bulb is also changed.

The skin appendages are also affected by age. The nails also change with ageing. They grow slower and may become dull and brittle. They may become yellow and opaque. Nails, particularly toenails, may become hard and thick. Ingrown toenails are more common. The tips of the fingernails may also fragment or split.

Hair loss does not decrease, but the hair follicles become less dense and less active. Hair colour changes as the follicle produces less melanin, hair loss occurs and the rate of hair growth changes. Many hair follicles stop producing hair altogether, and the remaining hair may become coarser. The dermal papillae flatten with the loss of the rete ridge, and this results in greater slippage between the epidermis and the dermis (skin tears occur more easily). Sweat glands and sebaceous glands are less dense and as such less productive; the result is seen as a decrease in the hydration of the skin.

Dermis

Assessment of an older person's skin may reveal that it is thin, fragile and inelastic. The rate at which fibroblasts reproduce decreases and this reduced production leads to a scant and poorer quality of collagen output. With the loss of blood vessels, there will be a marked reduction in the rate of neoangiogenesis (new blood vessel growth). These two features together mean slower rates of granulation tissue growth and also a poorer quality of granulation tissue. The blood vessels of the dermis become more fragile, this leads to bruising, bleeding under the skin (known as senile purpura), cherry angiomas and similar conditions. Raised collections of blood (haematomas) may form even after a minor injury.

Decreased elastin production results in decreased resilience of the skin, as well as the decreased resistance to external friction and shear forces. The ageing lymphatic system is less able to manage and maintain normal interstitial fluid levels.

Subcutaneous tissue

Consequences of a decrease in the amount of subcutaneous tissue are atrophy and fragile skin in an ageing person. Fragmenting of elastin results in the development of fibre networks forming fine wrinkles. Sensory perception is altered, giving rise to a decreased ability to discriminate between heat, pain, vibration and itching, putting that older person at an increased risk of injury.

The subcutaneous fat layer becomes thin, reducing normal insulation and padding. This increases the risk of skin injury and reduces a person's ability to maintain body temperature. As a result of the reduction in natural insulation, there is an increased risk of hypothermia in cold weather.

The fat layer absorbs some medications and the loss of the subcutaneous fat layer changes the way that these medications work. The use of patch medication may need to be reconsidered.

Skin changes and loss of subcutaneous fat combined with a tendency to be less active, as well as some nutritional deficiencies and other illnesses contribute to the development of pressure ulcers. Ageing skin repairs itself slower than younger skin. Wound-healing can be up to four times slower. This contributes to the development of pressure ulcers and infection. Diabetes, blood vessel changes, lowered immunity, and similar factors also affect healing.

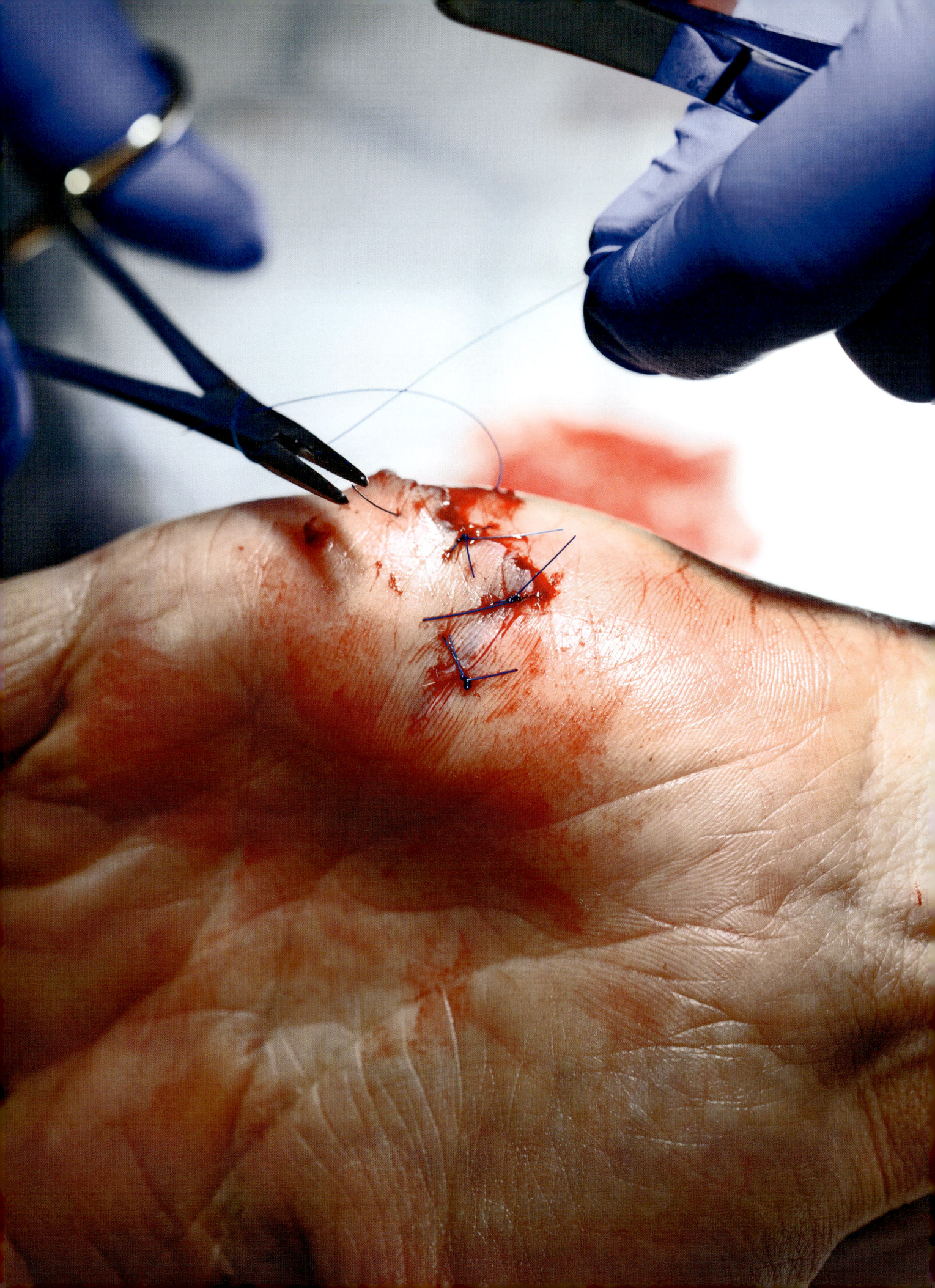

The normal healing process: acute wounds

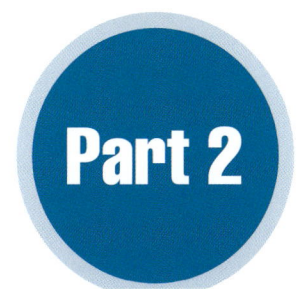

Part 2

Chapters

6	Haemostasis	16
7	Inflammation	18
8	Proliferation (granulation and epithelialisation)	20
9	Maturation	22
10	Factors affecting wound-healing	24

 Visit the companion website at **www.ataglanceseries.com/nursing/woundcare** to test yourself on these topics.

6 Haemostasis

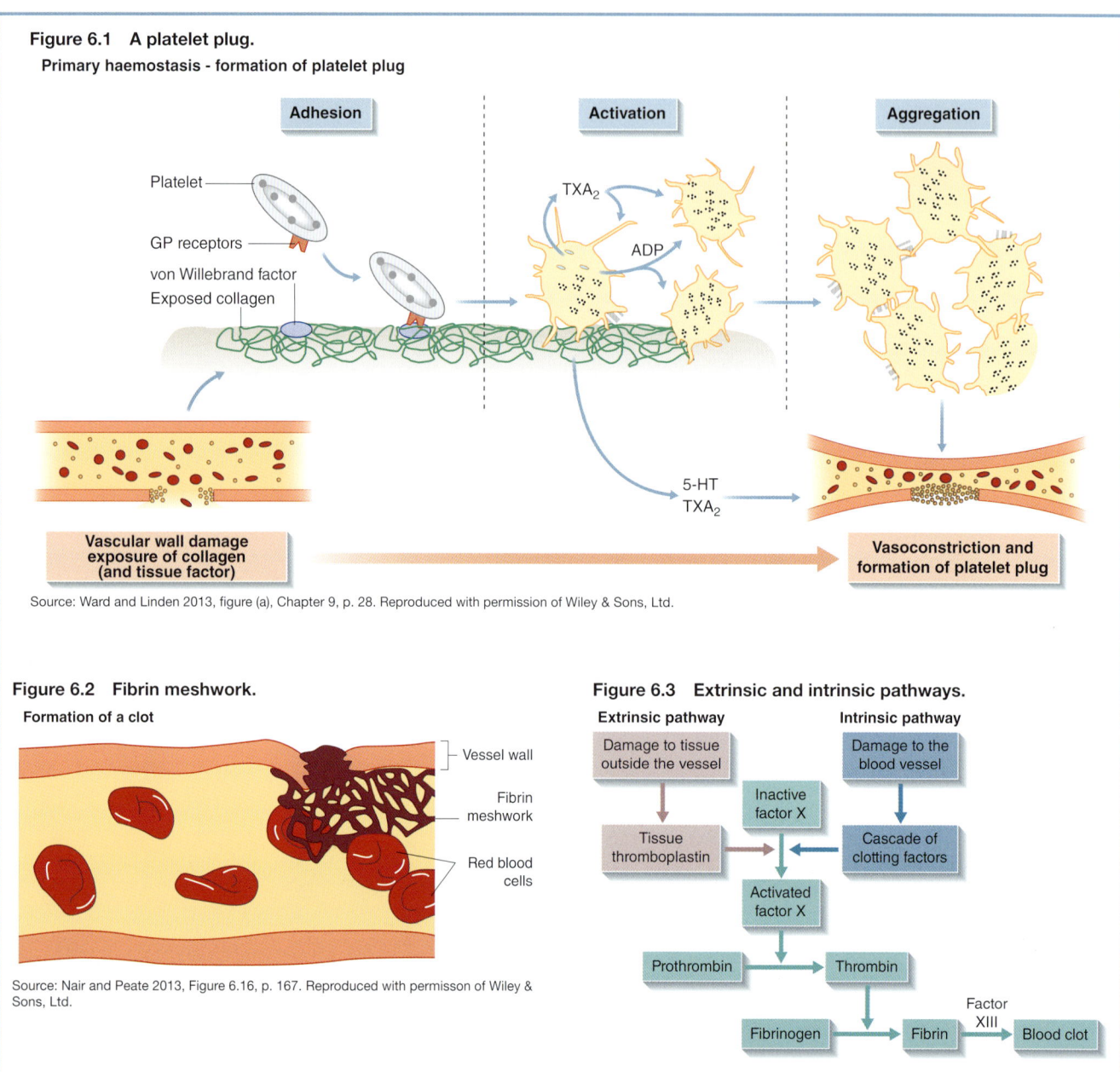

Figure 6.1 A platelet plug.
Figure 6.2 Fibrin meshwork.
Figure 6.3 Extrinsic and intrinsic pathways.

Physiology of haemostasis

The haemostatic mechanism is complex and delicately balanced. Haemostasis is an aspect of the wound-healing process. The wound-healing process passes through a number of phases, including inflammation, granulation and maturation.

Haemostasis is a process that causes bleeding to stop, keeping blood within a damaged blood vessel; the opposite of haemostasis is haemorrhage, and it is the first stage of wound-healing.

The body's initial response to wounding is to control the loss of blood from the area. Following damage to blood vessels and endothelial cells, platelets become sticky and adhere to the wall of the blood vessel and to each other, forming a platelet thrombus. The platelet thrombus acts as a temporary plug that reduces blood flow out of the wound (see Figure 6.1). The platelets also release serotonin and other chemical mediators, which results in a short period of vasoconstriction. Haemostasis is also achieved by the activation of the clotting cascade, initiated by damage to the endothelium.

Platelet function

Platelet function is essential in haemostasis. Platelets are vesicle-like fragments; they are incomplete cells, approximately 2–4 µm in diameter, discoid in shape and arise from larger cells, the megakaryocytes, in the bone marrow. The normal platelet count is approximately 150–400 million per millilitre of blood.

Five events occur when there is injury to a blood vessel:

1 Local vasoconstriction
2 Adhesion and aggregation of platelets
3 Activation of the clotting cascade
4 Activation of coagulation inhibitors
5 Fibrinolysis.

When damage to a blood vessel occurs, constriction occurs through direct action and also indirectly through the release of vasoconstrictors from platelets; these actions play a central role in limiting blood loss. Damage to the endothelial lining of the blood vessel also triggers platelet activity; when this happens, the platelets aggregate forming a plug. These actions along with the transient vasoconstriction are generally responsible for the cessation of bleeding. Platelets, when activated, also liberate a number of vasoconstrictor substances, revealing a phospholipid that is essential for the creation of a blood clot.

Generally, platelets do not adhere to the smooth endothelial lining of the blood vessels. However, when the vasculature is damaged, this exposes the blood to subendothelial collagen and microfibrils. The platelets stick to the collagen in the damaged vessel via glycoproteins (GPs) (von Willebrand factor enhances the adhesion) that are located on the surface of the platelets. Activation results in the platelets changing shape along with the production of pseudopodia (these are temporary protrusions), producing thromboxane A_2 (TXA_2) – an enzyme (a lipid with prothrombotic properties) – along with the release of 5-hydroxytryptamine (5-HT or serotonin) and ADP (adenosine diphosphate). Further vasoconstriction occurs caused by TXA_2 and 5-HT; ADP recruits more platelets and they aggregate to each other cross-linking with fibrinogen. A soft plug forms that is held together by fibrinogen molecules that create bridges between adjacent platelets. The aggregated platelets occlude the wound, which eventually stops bleeding. This is an unstable primary plug, a loosely aggregated plug, and has to be consolidated into a more stable plug.

Clotting cascade

The clotting cascade provides this more stable consolidated plug and ultimately results in the conversion of the plasma protein fibrinogen to fibrin, which forms a meshwork providing a seal to the damaged vasculature (see Figure 6.2). The cascade is a sequence of interactions between proteins that cause fibrin depositions at the location of tissue injury and is initiated by its interaction with activated factor VII. See Figure 6.3 for the extrinsic and intrinsic pathways.

The initial phase (this used to be known as the extrinsic pathway) involves several factors. Tissue factors VII and VIIa convert factor X to its active form, factor Xa. Tissue factor VIIa also converts factor IX to its activated form, factor IXa; further generation of factor Xa is inhibited by the tissue factor pathway inhibitor. At this point, the amount of factor Xa produced is insufficient to sustain coagulation. Further, factor Xa to allow haemostasis from progress to completion can now only be generated by the factor IXa pathway; by this stage though, enough thrombin has been generated by factor Xa to activate factors VIII and V. Both of these act as potent catalysts. Factor VIIIa increases the capacity of factor IXa to activate factor X to Xa many thousand times. The increased factor Xa produced in this way along with its own cofactor, activated Va, forms a complex that promotes the efficient conversion of prothrombin to thrombin. Thrombin then allows the conversion of fibrinogen to fibrin. The final result of the cascade is the production of fibrin, the biological glue that eventually seals the haemostatic plug ensuring haemostasis. As soon as a small amount of thrombin is formed, the clotting process accelerates and provides more and more thrombin into the wound. At high concentrations, this thrombin quickly converts fibrinogen to fibrin on the surface of the platelet aggregate to stabilise the haemostatic plug. Over the course of the subsequent 7–12 days, the process of fibrinolysis dissolves the fibrin in the wound, as the site of injury heals and the cell layer in the vessel wall is restored. Scar formation occurs, and the wound is completely healed within a few weeks.

Wound healing

Wound healing is a complex and dynamic process that varies according to the location and type of wound and occurs as a systemic process, which follows in stepwise fashion and involves the stages of haemostasis, inflammation and repair. Generally, from injury to resolution, wounds go through four phases:

1 Haemostasis
2 Inflammation
3 Proliferation
4 Remodelling.

As the fibrin formation occurs, a protective wound scab is formed. Scab formation provides a surface beneath which cell migration and movement of the wound edges can follow. The inflammatory process brings nutrients to the area of the wound, removes debris and bacteria and makes chemical stimuli available to start the wound repair. Repair begins instantaneously after wounding and proceeds quickly through the processes of epithelialisation, fibroplasia and capillary proliferation into the healing area. Different tissues possess their own normal rates of growth as the healing process occurs. The ideal rate of healing happens when there are factors present that are advantageous to healing, and the factors that have the ability to disturb or hinder the healing processes are controlled or absent.

7 Inflammation

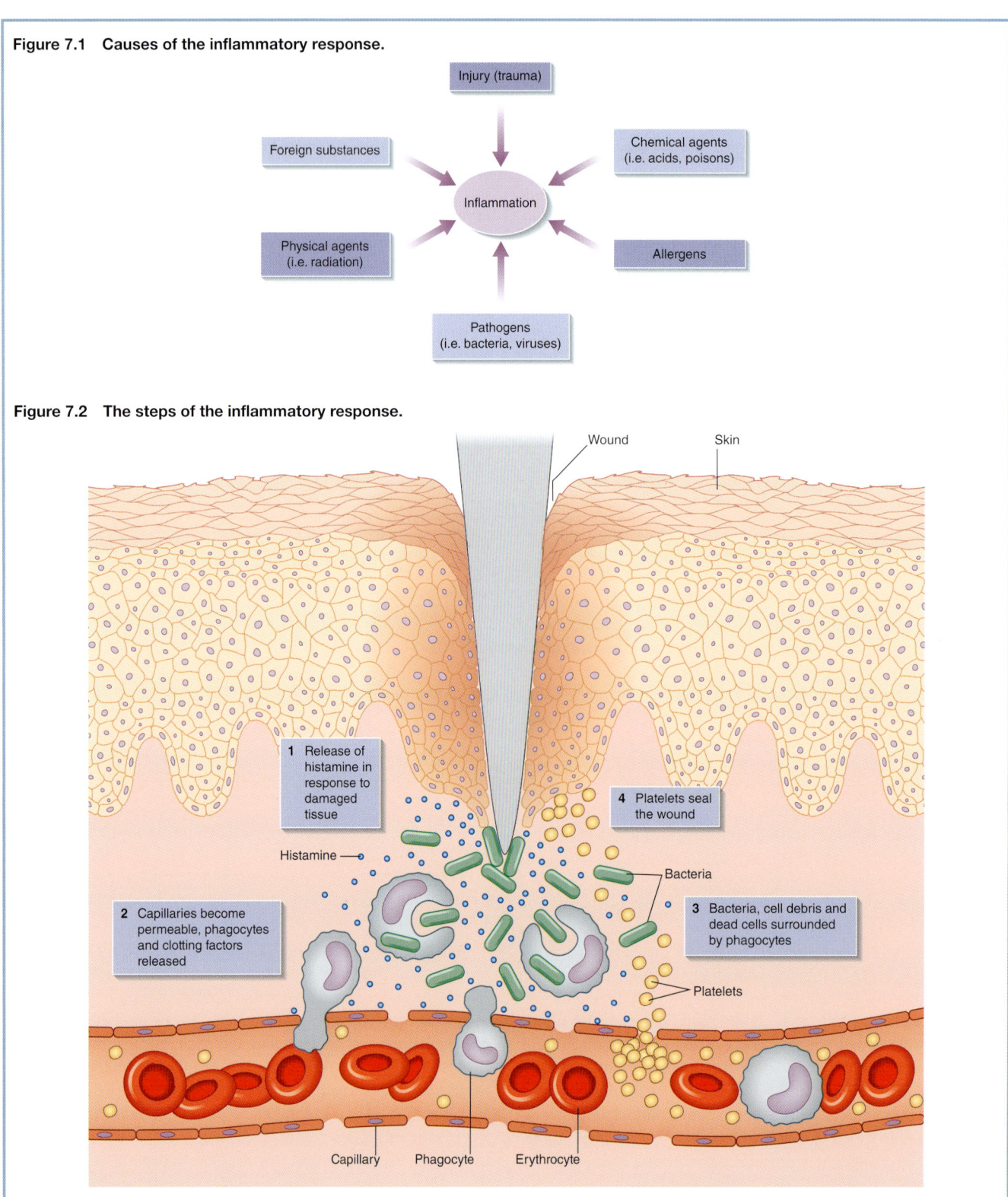

Figure 7.1 Causes of the inflammatory response.

Figure 7.2 The steps of the inflammatory response.

Wound Care at a Glance, Second Edition. Ian Peate and Melanie Stephens.
© 2020 John Wiley & Sons Ltd. Published 2020 by John Wiley & Sons Ltd.
Companion website: http://www.ataglanceseries.com/nursing/woundcare/

Inflammation

When there is an insult to the body, for example, a trauma or any intentional injury resulting in damage to the blood vessels, the first response is to arrest the haemorrhage. The prevention of blood loss and the formation of clots and scabs are the parts of the haemostatic process in an attempt to provide a protective covering when the skin is broken.

The body has effective mechanisms to block potential pathogens from entering the body, including the skin and mucous membranes as physical barriers. Enzymes, such as lysozymes in tears and sweat, have the capacity to destroy many potential pathogens chemically; however, even with these external barriers available to fight potential pathogens, there are occasions when pathogens enter the body. When this occurs and infection is present, the body sets the inflammatory response into action. This response is non-specific and attacks any and all foreign invaders. This inflammatory response is a universal reaction to tissue damage. See Figure 7.1 for the causes of the inflammatory response.

The inflammation attempts to rid the body of microbes, toxins or other foreign material at the site of injury with the intention of preventing their spread to other tissues; it also begins to prepare the site for tissue repair.

The inflammatory response

Inflammation is an innate response to tissue damage, with four phases (or characteristic signs) associated with the inflammatory response:

1 Redness (rubor)
2 Swelling (tumour)
3 Heat (calor)
4 Pain (dolor).

Loss of function is the fifth phase added to the original four. Inflammation can result in a loss of function; for example, the inability to detect sensation depending on the site and extent of the injury.

In case of an injury, pathogens such as bacteria, virus or fungus gain entry into the body. Almost immediately, a number of events are caused by the damaged cells, such as:

1 Vasodilation
2 Messenger molecules are released
3 Activation of complement
4 Extravasation of vascular components
5 Phagocytosis
6 Pain.

The injured mast cells in the connective tissue release histamine. The arrival of histamine at the site of injury has an immediate impact on blood vessels in the region. Arterioles dilate and venules constrict, causing an increase in blood flow. Vasodilation is brought about by four main mechanisms.

1 The kinin system in the cell produces bradykinin, a vasodilator, which is also responsible for pain.
2 Damaged plasma membranes release arachidonic acid, a fatty acid and a precursor to prostaglandins. Prostaglandins are also vasodilators and have hyperalgesic properties (they increase pain).
3 Release of histamine from the degranulated mast cells increases the pore size between the capillary cells, permitting movement of proteins and other micromolecules into interstitial spaces.
4 Vascular epithelial cells release nitric oxide, a vasodilator. Macrophages also release large amounts of nitric oxide.

Increased blood flow explains the redness and heat associated with the infection. Capillaries within injured tissue dilate, becoming permeable; this is essential for an appropriate inflammatory response, providing an opportunity for some of the blood components to be released into the damaged area and the site of infection (Figure 7.2).

Platelets and clotting factors

Platelets and their associated clotting factors (see Chapter 6) (for example, thrombin and fibrinogen) exit through the leaky capillary walls and migrate towards the site of injury. The clotting factors serve a dual purpose when this occurs; they help to plug the wound and seal damaged blood vessels; they also confine infectious agents to the wound site slowing their systemic spread.

Chemokines

A second line of defence also becomes activated. Cells close to the injury release a series of chemical signals radiating from the site of inflammation; these signals are known as chemokines. A very high concentration of chemokines immediately surrounds the infection. High levels of chemokines attract or provide a signal for the attraction of phagocytic white blood cells including the neutrophils.

Phagocytosis

As the chemokine concentration continues to increase, phagocytes leave the capillary entering the site of infection and macrophages arrive 24 hours later. Phagocytes engulf and destroy the present pathogens, recognising the pathogen as a non-self-matter and sending out the pseudopodia surrounding the pathogen. The wound site begins to heal. After the white blood cells engulf the pathogen particles, they begin to die; they eventually form the pus associated with infected cuts. The key molecule released is interleukin 1, attracting neutrophils and macrophages to the site of injury and helping to clear away debris from the injured area.

Phagocytosis results in a metabolically intensive activity and is responsible for some of the heat associated with inflammation. Pyrexia occurs during infection accompanying the inflammation. Bacterial toxins elevate the body temperature, releasing cytokines from macrophages causing the increase in temperature. The presence of pyrexia exaggerates the impact of interferons, hindering the growth of some microbes speeding up the reactions that aid repair.

When the pathogen particles are destroyed and the damaged tissue is repaired, histamine signals fade and blood vessels return to their normal size.

The sensation of pain in inflammation is increased by the action and interaction of bradykinin and prostaglandins. Other chemicals are also involved in the stimulation of pain after the injury; lactic acid produced by anaerobic cellular respiration is one example. Hydrogen ions and potassium released from damaged cells also stimulate the pain receptors.

Inflammation lasts for approximately 4–5 days. The process requires energy and nutritional resources for efficacy. With large complex wounds, demands made on the body are considerable. Inflammation has a protective function helping to eliminate the cause(s) of tissue damage. Extending the inflammatory stage – for example, where there is infection, the presence of a foreign body or damage that has been caused by an inappropriate dressing – can have an adverse effect on the person's health and well-being.

8 Proliferation (granulation and epithelialisation)

Figure 8.1 Wound-healing time scales.

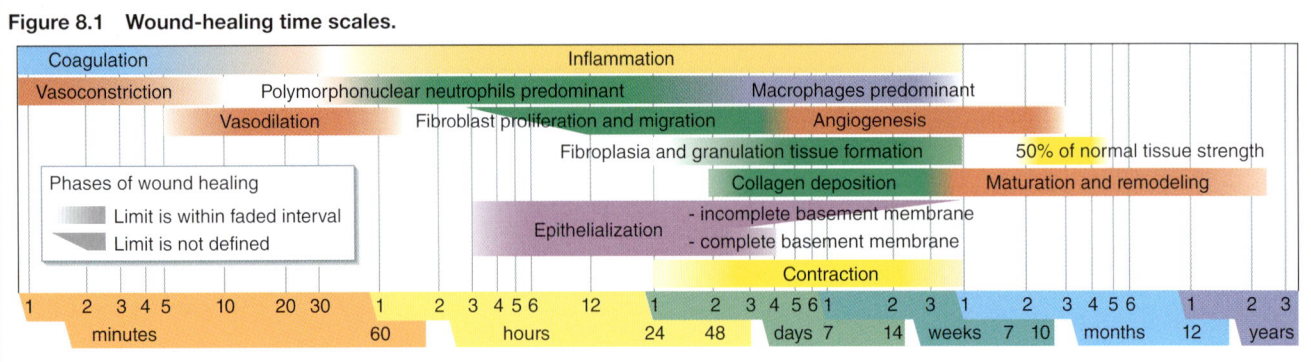

Figure 8.2 Proliferative phase of wound-healing showing fibroblasts producing extracellular matrix and re-epithelialisation by keratinocytes.

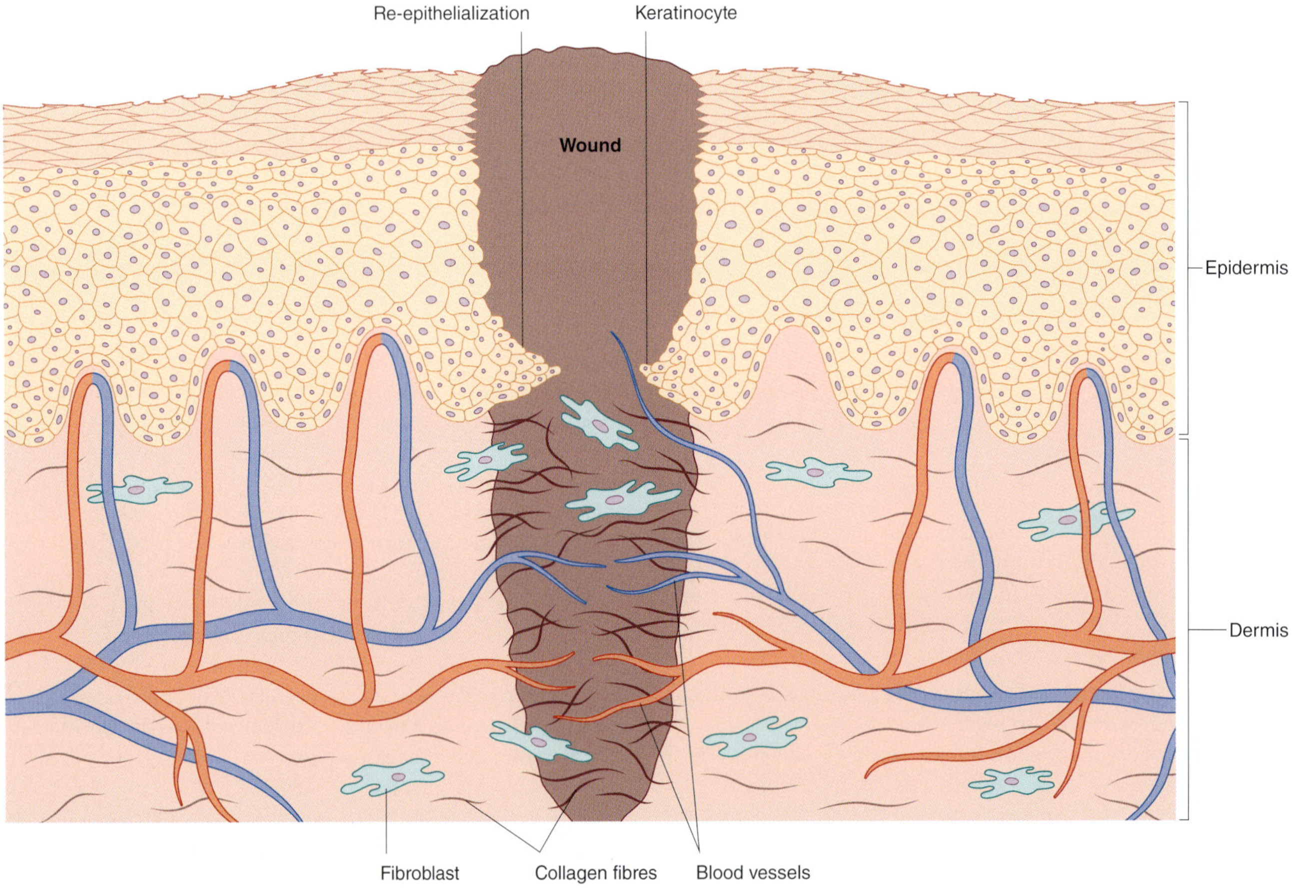

Wound-healing consists of filling the gap created by tissue destruction followed by restoration of the structural continuity of the injured part through three phases of healing (Figure 8.1); they are:

1 The inflammatory phase
2 The proliferative phase
3 The remodelling phase.

Proliferation

The proliferation phase overlaps with the inflammation stage (see Chapter 7), as this phase starts to end. The focus of the proliferative phase is associated with the building of new tissue to fill the wound space. As the inflammation diminishes, the process to repair the injury starts. About 3 days after the injury, fibroblasts start to enter and assemble in the wound; this is the start of the transition from inflammatory phase to proliferation phase. The fibroblasts are the connective tissue cells that synthesise and secrete collagen. The secretion of growth factors that induce the growth of blood vessels starts through the process of angiogenesis along with promoting endothelial cell proliferation and migration. As the fibroblasts grow and form, they produce a new, provisional extracellular matrix that comes about by excreting collagen and fibronectin.

The fibroblasts and endothelial cells form granulation tissue that acts as the foundation for scar tissue development (Figure 8.2).

Granulation

Granulation tissue contains newly developed capillary buds. Granulation tissue can be seen in the wound around the end of the first week; this tissue continues to grow until the wound is healed. This tissue is rich in new blood vessels and other components that are required to fill in the injured tissue. Granulation tissue is usually bright red or pink, moist, soft in touch and has a bumpy appearance, it is fragile and bleeds easily. The masses within the injured tissue keep growing and contracting depending on the wound type; this takes approximately 8 weeks for a standard open healing excision wound and 4 weeks for a closed (sutured) wound.

Around day 5 post injury, exudate appears in the wound (this is the by-product of healing and is a sticky greenish-white substance resembling pus, but is not). If too much exudate is produced, wound healing may be slowed; increased exudate may be an indication of infection and increased oedema.

Epithelialisation, maturation and remodelling

The final feature of the proliferative stage is epithelialisation; this is the regeneration, migration, proliferation and differentiation of epithelial cells at the wound's edge forming a new surface area similar to that destroyed by the injury. Just after the injury, cytokines are released from platelets and they activate keratinocytes. As the migration of keratinocytes occurs, re-epithelialisation begins as early as 2 hours after wounding. Growth factors, such as keratinocytes growth factor (KGF) and epidermal growth factor (EGF), provoke the proliferation and migration of keratinocytes. The main sources of migrating keratinocytes during re-epithelialisation process are basal keratinocytes from the wound edges, dermal appendages, such as hair follicles, sweat and sebaceous glands and bone marrow–derived keratinocyte stem cells. Keratinocytes secrete proteases and plasminogen activator that activates plasmin. Migration of keratinocytes over the wound site is also enhanced by the lack of contact inhibition and the release of nitric oxide from polymorphonuclear leucocytes (PMNs), keratinocytes and fibroblasts. Epithelial cells continue migrating across the wound bed until cells from different sides meet in the middle; at this point, the contact between keratinocytes inhibits further migration. New layers of keratinocytes differentiate, and this gives rise to a stratified epidermis.

As the proliferative stage ends, white bloods cells leave the area and oedema diminishes; the wound begins to blanch as the small blood vessels begin to thrombose and degenerate.

The maturation and remodelling phases overlap with the proliferation phase, as the healing begins to come to an end. The remodelling phase begins after about 3 weeks and can continue for 6 months or longer. Final scar tissue starts to form by the simultaneous synthesis of lysis and collagen. Collagen is fibrous in character, and connects and supports tissues and organs, such as skin, bone, tendons, muscles and cartilage. It is often referred to as the glue that holds the body together; it is collagen that provides tensile strength. There are over 25 types of collagen that occur naturally in the body; collagen can be found both inside and outside cells, contributing to the structure of cells.

At this stage, the process of remodelling of the collagen fibres is laid down. The scar becomes avascular.

The wound is made smaller by the action of myofibroblasts, as the edges of the wound are drawn closer together. This establishes a grip on the edges of the wound, causing them to contract using a mechanism that is similar to that in smooth muscle cells. When the role of myofibroblasts is close to completion, cells that are no longer needed undergo apoptosis. Myofibroblastic activity can persist, contributing to fibrosis and scarring in the skin.

Nerve endings now start to redevelop, and the tissue starts to rearrange itself. The scar tissue may achieve 70–80% of tensile strength by the end of 3 months. Within the tissue, there is much physiological activity left even after the surface wound-healing. This final phase continues for up to 18 months after the wound is closed.

Rapid keratinocyte migration along with re-epithelialisation can often lead to better wound-healing outcomes and decreased scar formation. However, exposure to air and/or lack of moisture will result in a delay in the healing process.

This whole process is complex, and the skin is fragile and prone to interruption or failure. The outcome of this is the formation of non-healing chronic wounds. There are factors that may contribute to the interruption or failure, such as:

- Diabetes
- Venous or arterial disease
- Infection
- Ageing.

9 Maturation

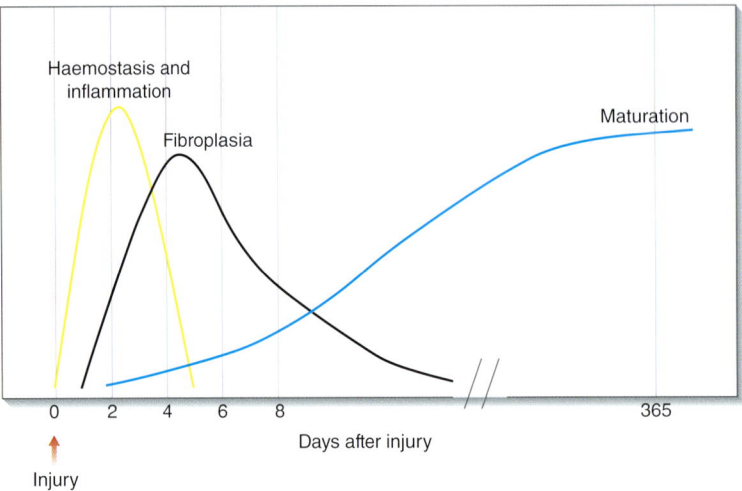

Figure 9.1 The phases of wound-healing.

Box 9.1 Wound–healing.

- The stages of wound-healing are complex.
- This is a fragile process.
- Failure to progress in the stage of wound-healing has the potential to lead to chronic wounds.
- Careful, patient-centred wound care can accelerate the wound-healing process.

Wound healing

This text explains that there are many factors associated with the healing of wounds, for example, internal (coexisting disease, the ageing process and nutritional status) and external (pressure, friction and sheer) factors. Wound-healing is a natural response to the tissue injury, a restorative response. Healing occurs as a result of the interaction of a complex cascade of cellular events that produces resurfacing, reconstitution and restoration of the tensile strength of the skin that has been injured. There are also a number of phases of wound healing (Figure 9.1):

- The vascular response (this is where haemostasis takes place)
- The inflammatory response (here the body puts in place a variety of inflammatory responses)
- The proliferation phase (the active growth phase with granulation and epithelisation occurring)
- The maturation phase.

Whilst healing is a systematic process, the four classic phases mentioned above often overlap with each other (as is the case here). For the sake of discussion and understanding, the process of wound- healing is usually presented as a series of separate discrete events. In reality, it must be noted that the whole process is much more complicated, as cellular events that lead to scar formation overlap. There are many aspects of wound-healing that are still to be understood.

The maturation phase

Collagen

During the maturation phase, collagen remodelling depends on the continued collagen synthesis in the presence of collagen destruction. In the wound, collagenases and matrix metalloproteinases (an enzyme) help with the removal of excess collagen, as the synthesis of new collagen persists. Tissue inhibitors of metalloproteinases limit these collagenolytic enzymes, helping ensure that a balance exists between the creation of new collagen and the elimination of old collagen.

As the remodelling occurs, collagen becomes more progressively organised. A number of complex interactions take place with fibronectin gradually disappearing and hyaluronic acid and glycosaminoglycans replaced by proteoglycans. The types of collagen change, and type III collagen is replaced by type I collagen. Water is resorbed from the scar. These events allow the collagen fibres to lie closer together, enabling collagen cross-linking and ultimately reducing scar thickness. Intramolecular and intermolecular collagen cross-links result in increased wound bursting strength (tensile strength). Approximately 21 days after injury, the remodelling begins when the net collagen content of the wound is stable; this can continue indefinitely. Wound-healing is a complex process; see Box 9.1 for details.

The measurement of the tensile strength of a wound is its load capacity per unit area. The bursting strength of a wound is associated with the force needed to break a wound regardless of its dimension. Bursting strength differs according to skin thickness. The peak tensile strength of the wound is achieved approximately 60 days after the injury. When the wound heals, it only reaches approximately 80% of the tensile strength of the unwounded skin.

Cytokines

These are the significant mediators of wound-healing events. A cytokine is a protein mediator that is released from numerous cell sources, binding to cell surface receptors with the purpose of stimulating a cell response.

Cytokines can reach their target cell via various routes. The first cytokine described was the epidermal growth factor, which is a potent mitogen (a substance that encourages cell division) for epithelial cells, endothelial cells and fibroblasts. Epidermal growth factor stimulates other activities in the wound-healing factors, such as fibronectin synthesis, angiogenesis, fibroplasia and collagenase activity. Fibroblast growth factor stimulates angiogenesis. This factor also stimulates wound contraction, epithelialisation and the production of collagen.

Platelet derivative growth factor (PDGF) is released from the platelets and is responsible for the stimulation of neutrophils and macrophages. It is a mitogen and chemotactic agent for fibroblasts and smooth muscle cells, stimulating angiogenesis, collagen synthesis and collagenase.

Transforming growth factor-β is an important stimulant for fibroblast proliferation and the production of proteoglycans, collagen and fibrin. The factor promotes accumulation of the extracellular matrix and fibrosis; it has the ability to reduce scarring and to reverse the inhibition of wound-healing.

Tumour necrosis factor-α is produced by macrophages and stimulates angiogenesis and the synthesis of collagen and collagenase. This factor is a mitogen for fibroblasts.

During the maturation phase (also known as the 'reconstruction phase'), remodelling of the scar continues for approximately 1 year. Scar tissue regains about two-thirds of its original strength; it will never be as strong as the original tissue it replaces. Maturation is the final phase occurring once the wound is closed. This phase includes the remodelling of collagen from type III to type I. Cellular activity reduces, and the number of blood vessels in the wounded area regress and decrease.

The ability to closely approximate uninjured tissue is very much dependent on the size, depth, location and type of wound, as well as on a person's nutritional status, wound care and overall health.

10 Factors affecting wound-healing

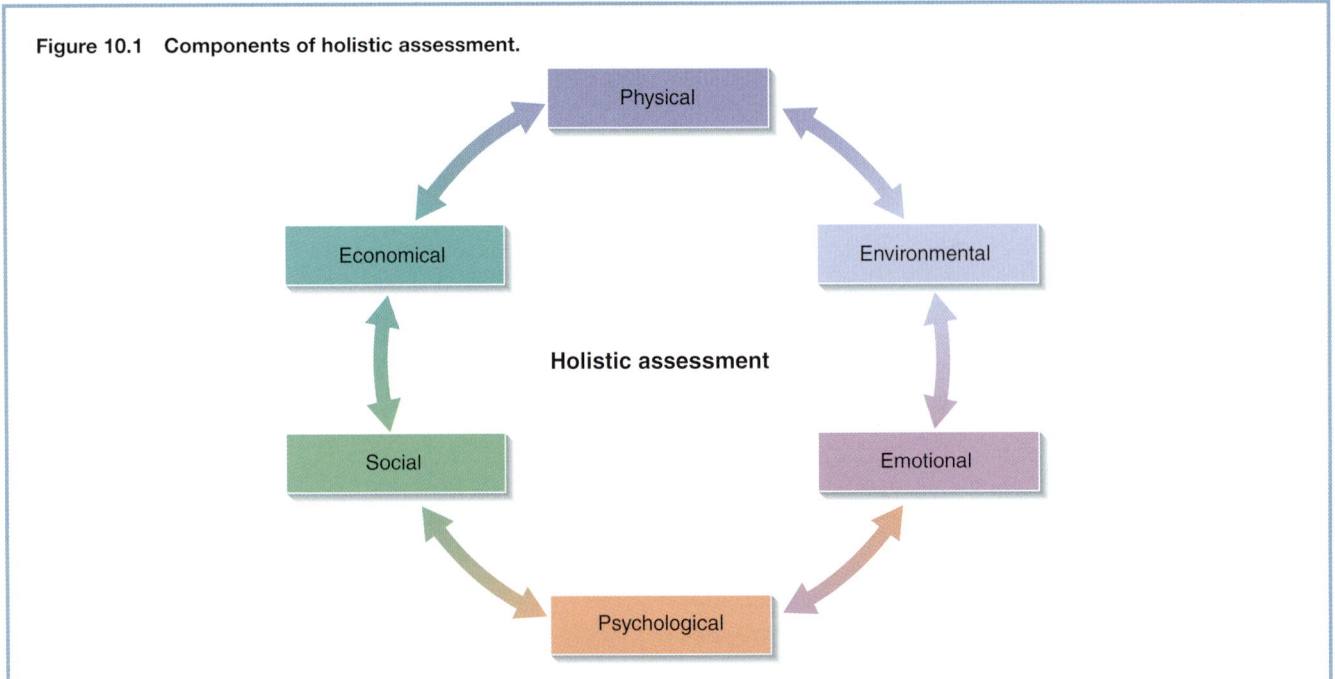

Figure 10.1 Components of holistic assessment.

Holistic assessment

There are many factors that influence the healing process and healing rates of wounds; these include physical, environmental, emotional, psychological, social and economical factors. In order to ensure that a wound progresses, as far as it is possible, through the normal healing process within a reasonable time frame, it is essential that these factors are considered when carrying out a wound assessment. Simply assessing the wound in isolation will not identify any issues that may be preventing a wound from healing, or which could be slowing down the rate at which it will heal. Therefore, a holistic assessment must be completed as regularly as a wound assessment in order to identify and rectify potential delays in the wound-healing rates. The holistic and wound assessment process will be discussed later in Chapter 17, and, in the meantime, Figure 10.1 shows how each factor can impact the other factors. Let us briefly consider some of these factors and how they can affect the patient and healing rates.

Physical

This factor considers the patient in the physical sense; for example, age, gender, underlying medical conditions, medications, physique, weight, height and lifestyle. In other words, all intrinsic factors associated with the patient. The failure to identify and address relevant physical issues, where it is possible to address them, could not only impact on the wounds' ability to heal but also on the following holistic issues.

Many aspects of the patient cannot be altered, such as age; however certain medical conditions, could be controlled to optimise the patient's health and healing prospects, such as diabetes.

Environmental

External factors can impact on a wound's ability to heal; therefore, consideration must be given to this aspect when assessing the patient; for example, the environment the patient is nursed in. It is important to consider who (if anyone) is providing care to the patient. Is the care appropriate? Are the staff/carer knowledgeable about the standards of care? Is the patient's clothing or footwear appropriate and not ill-fitting? Ill-fitted clothing could reduce circulation or add pressure to the patient's skin, resulting in wound deterioration or pressure damage. Is the surface on which the patient is sitting or lying comfortable? Are the medical devices that are being used safe enough? Surfaces and devices can easily cause pressure damage or affect the circulation of blood to a wound, if kept in the same vicinity. Is the patient getting access to good nutrition? Who is providing the food, and is it of good quality? The environment as a whole must be considered when assessing the patient (more on this later).

The wound environment must be considered a priority. There is always the possibility of an inappropriate dressing applied to a wound that does not maintain a moist wound-healing environment that is conducive to optimum healing. Also, if wound dressings are being tampered with by the patient or by others (such as family, carers and other untrained, unskilled persons). These factors should be addressed and dealt with.

Emotional

What is affecting the patient's feelings? Is the patient worried about issues such as income? Does the patient have family worries or stressors? Does the patient have any kind of pain or anything else that could affect his/her emotions, such as bereavement or loneliness? Emotional issues are known to impact on the patient's physical well-being and skin integrity, and this can be evidenced in some people who are prone to developing rashes or herpes simplex (cold sores) when under a lot of emotional strain.

Psychological

This factor can be linked quite closely with the symptoms resulting from emotions, which can impact on the patient's psychological status and can lead to psychological breakdown. It is important to consider factors such as psychological illness and neurological impairments, such as dementia, all of which could affect the patient's mental capacity (either permanent or temporary). Psychological issues can impact on the patient's physical well-being in a similar way to any emotional burdens they may have, whilst exacerbating those emotions.

Social

The examples of social issues could be loneliness and isolation, poor housing and/or living conditions, poor nutrition, poor standards in hygiene, overcrowding and lifestyle. This factor can also be linked to emotional and psychological status of a patient, and if left unaddressed could impact on their physical well-being. For example, a patient with a malodorous wound could become isolated due to the embarrassment about the odour emanating from their wound. In time, the patient could become housebound, lose their independence and become lonely due to the lack of socialising.

Economical

This factor could indicate financial issues with the patient that could impact on the type and quality of nutrition the person is able to afford. The cost issue with regard to the lack of appropriate bedding, seating, clothing or footwear could impact on the patient's wound and skin integrity as a whole. This factor could also have a bearing on all of the aforementioned factors.

The type of dressing must also be considered for use on the wound; whilst cost-effectiveness must always be aimed for, it is not always the case that the cheapest or most expensive product is the most appropriate.

Whilst cost must be a consideration in all of the above economical aspects, much of it is out of the control of the nurse and may be dependent on the patient's own budget. However, where possible, due consideration must be given to the patient's needs, and finance must not be the main driving force when selecting any products or devices.

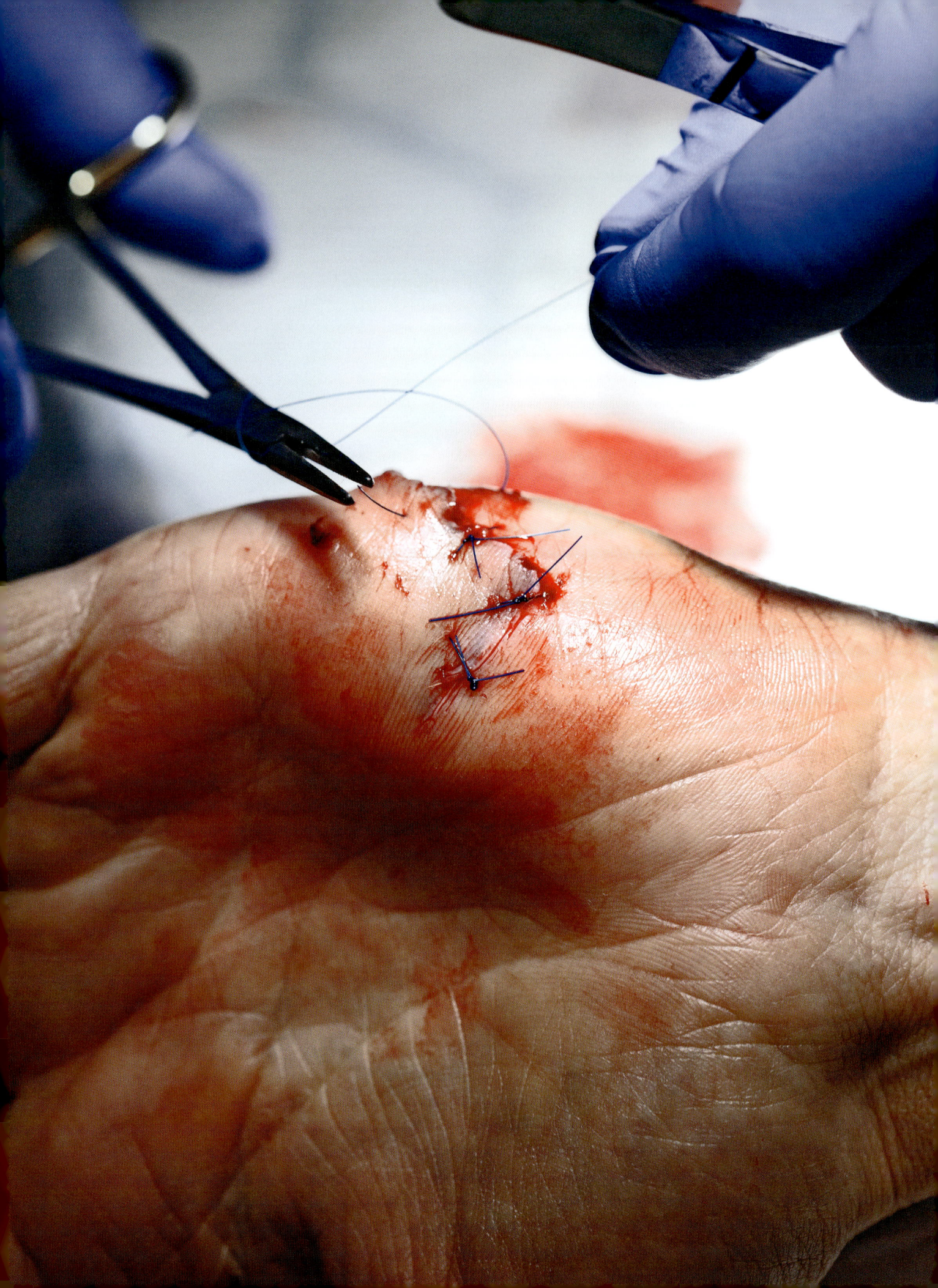

The abnormal healing process: chronic wound healing

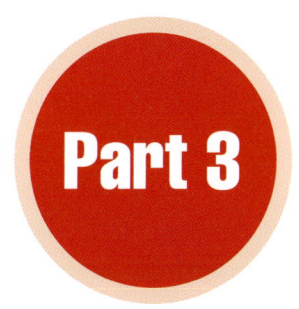

Part 3

Chapters

11	The impaired healing process	28
12	Factors affecting wound-healing	30
13	Nutrition and wound-healing	32
14	Incontinence and wounds	34
15	Vascular disease	36

 Visit the companion website at www.ataglanceseries.com/nursing/woundcare to test yourself on these topics.

11 The impaired healing process

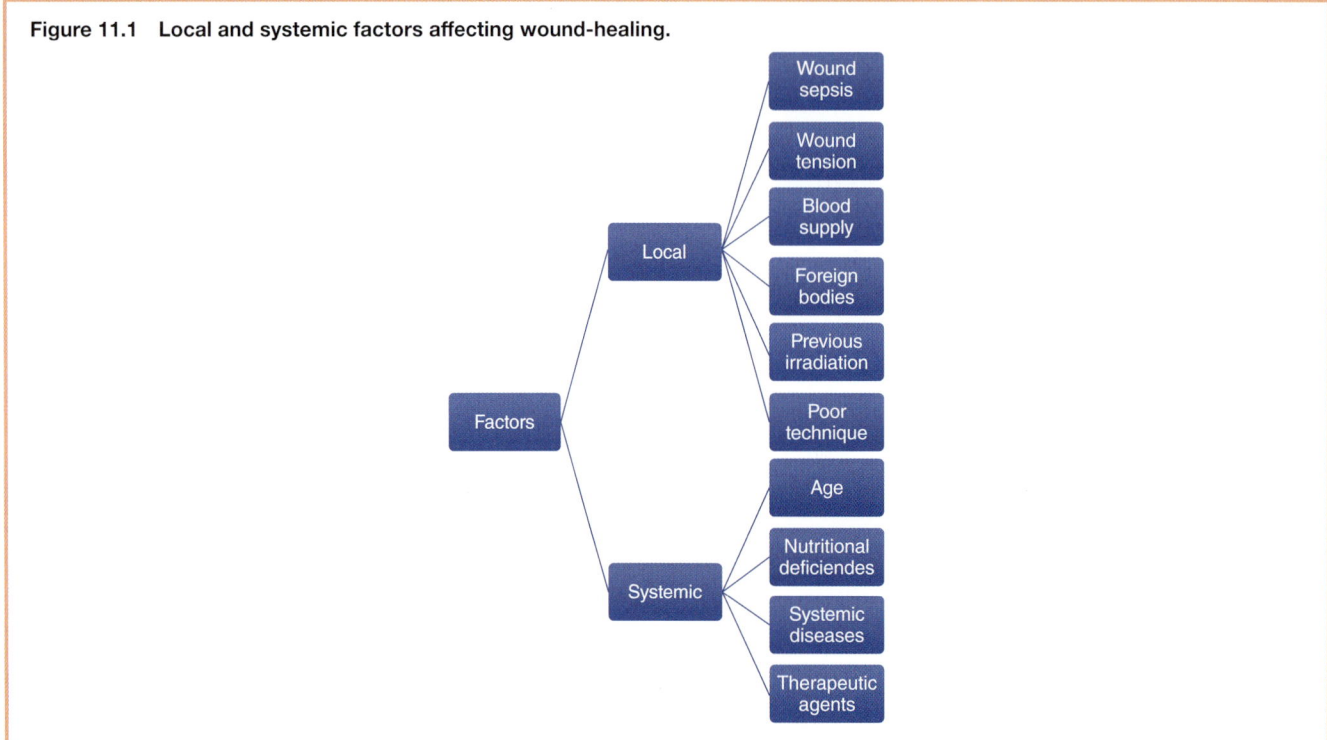

Figure 11.1 Local and systemic factors affecting wound-healing.

Factors that affect the healing process can be intrinsic (for example, age, gender, allergies), extrinsic (such as clothing, footwear, bed, chair) or both (i.e. intrinsic and extrinsic) (see Figure 11.1). Let us now look at these factors and consider how they can hinder the normal healing process that we have already discussed in the previous chapters. In this chapter, we will also consider how these intrinsic and extrinsic factors can be managed in order to promote a wound to progress through the normal phases of healing within a reasonable timescale.

Considering both intrinsic and extrinsic factors, the four phases of wound-healing and the potential reasons that could affect this process are:

1 *Haemostasis*: The wound does not stop bleeding within 5–10 minutes of the injury, even after applying pressure. The cause of continued bleeding may be a severed large blood vessel; a clotting disorder, for example, low platelets (thrombocytopaenia) or haemophilia; or the patient taking anticoagulant medications, such as aspirin or warfarin. If the wound does not reach haemostasis (with firm pressure) within 10–20 minutes, the patient requires immediate medical assistance.

2 *Inflammatory response*: There are two potential ways to interrupt this response.
   (a) A wound may not enter this phase due to the patient taking anti-inflammatory medication (which reduces the flow of the blood supply to the wound bed); or there may be a severely reduced blood supply, whereby white blood cells (e.g. phagocytes) do not reach the site of the injury. In any of these events, the wound will either heal slowly or not at all through this phase. During this time, the wound is at a greater risk of infection due to the lack of essential white cells reaching the wound bed.
   (b) A patient may have an inflammatory condition, for example, rheumatoid arthritis, ulcerative colitis or Crohn's disease, and if their condition is in "flare up" when the person has a wound, then it is probable that the wound will enter and remain in this phase. This means that the wound will be unable to progress to healing, and it will be vulnerable to infection as the levels of bacteria on the wound bed increase over time.

3 *Regenerative phase*: This is the most common phase for delays in wound-healing and is usually the result of one of the extrinsic factors, such as incorrect dressing choices, poor dressing technique and poor exudate management. For example, if a dressing is allowed to adhere to a wound, it will cause trauma to the wound bed on dressing removal, and so the wound has to once again go through the inflammatory response, thereby delaying wound-healing by up to 5 days. Similarly, if a dressing is allowed to become saturated, migrating granulation and epithelial cells will become macerated and will be destroyed, and, as a result healing will not take place. The longer a wound takes to heal, the more likely it becomes infected, as the bioburden increases on the wound bed over time.

4 *Maturation phase*: This is the 'shrinking' phase of wound-healing whereby the collagen and elastic fibre matrix reorganise in order to increase the tensile strength of the scar tissue. This process continues throughout the healing process in symmetry with the regenerative phase and continues for many years after the wound is completely re-epithelialised.

As the tissues shrink, contractures can occur, particularly over the palm of hands, face and joints; this can restrict movement. Occasionally, keloid and hypertrophic scaring can occur, with poor cosmetic results. Often, massage can reduce these effects of abnormal maturation of tissues by assisting with the redistribution of collagen and elastic fibres. Occasionally, plastic surgeons recommend the use of silicone creams and dressings to reduce the effects of scarring and contractures; however, the evidences behind the efficacy of these products to date are limited.

While some of the factors that hinder the healing rates for a given individual are uncontrollable, others are not, and it is therefore essential that the nurse responsible for assessing, treating and managing a patient with a wound carries out a holistic assessment that considers both extrinsic and intrinsic factors before deciding on the most appropriate method for the treatment of any wound. This is rather like a prescriber prescribing a drug; the prescriber ensures that they are fully aware of any comorbidities and the medications the person is taking before prescribing something new. The formal assessment process must therefore consider the following before treating the wound:

1 *Extrinsic factors* (this list is not exhaustive): Clothing, footwear, bed, chair, home environment, lifestyle, dressing choice, nurse's/carer's knowledge and expertise in wound management, patient knowledge and compliance, nutrition, socioeconomic status, and so forth.
2 *Intrinsic factors* (this list is not exhaustive): Age, gender, comorbidities, allergies, medications, skin type, scarring, nutrition, incontinence and immobility.
3 *Finally, the wound assessment must consider*: Dimensions, depth, peri-wound skin condition, exudate levels, tissue type and signs of infection (to be discussed later).

12 Factors affecting wound-healing

This chapter considers the factors that affect would healing from a chronic wound health perspective (also see Chapter 10). There are many reasons why wounds do not heal in a simple manner; these reasons can be classified as intrinsic (something internal to the individual) or extrinsic (something external to the individual). In some cases, these factors may be both intrinsic as well as extrinsic, as this chapter will explain. It is vital that the patient be assessed holistically, so that the factors influencing delayed healing rates can be identified and addressed as far as possible, after which the wound itself can be assessed. The following are some common factors that impact on wound-healing rates and should be considered during assessment. Many of the factors mentioned below have been discussed in greater detail in other chapters.

Intrinsic factors

- *Age*: As we age, cell regeneration rates slow down, which means that wounds usually take longer to heal with ageing. A wound that might take 3 weeks to heal in a younger person may take 6 weeks to heal in an older person. It is therefore important to set realistic goals when planning wound care.
- *Gender*: The fluctuating hormone levels in females during their lifetime appear to affect skin integrity, and, therefore, the healing rates, albeit in a minor way.
- *Psychological*: The psychological state can impact on wound healing, such as high levels of emotional stress, worry and negative thought processes. Evidence of this can be seen where a person develops a mouth ulcer or cold sores when he/she experiences such emotional pressures.
- *Physical/structure*: The human body structure itself can be a factor in wound-healing rates, and one example of this is where pressure ulcers exist; the underlying bone that caused the ulcer in the first instance will continue to delay wound healing if pressure relief is not ensured. Other physical factors that must be considered are, for example, scar tissue, physical deformities, particularly of limbs, amputations, mobility and reduced mobility.
- *Lifestyle*: Smoking, alcoholism and drug use, although extrinsic factors, can impact intrinsically on the individual, which could delay healing rates.
- *Nutrition*: This can be both an intrinsic factor (e.g. due to malabsorption conditions or gastric surgery) and an extrinsic factor (due to dietary choices), which can result in poor nutritional intake. As wound-healing requires increased nutritional intake, any reduction in this will impact on healing rates.
- *Medications*: Common medications that impact on wound-healing processes and rates are steroids, anti-inflammatory drugs and cytotoxic drugs.
- *Comorbidities*: Common medical conditions that affect wound-healing rates are:
  - Diabetes, peripheral artery disease and other conditions that affect the blood circulation (such as heart disease and hypertension) mean that a reduced blood supply reaches the wound bed.
  - An inefficient cardiopulmonary circulation due to heart or lung disease means that the wound will receive a reduced supply of essential oxygen and nutrients that will reduce healing rates.
  - Inflammatory diseases, such as rheumatoid arthritis and ulcerative colitis; these conditions affect the inflammatory phase of wound healing if the condition flares up, which can cause a prolonged inflammatory phase. Alternatively, if the condition is in remission, the patient is usually taking prescribed steroids, which also delay the healing process by delaying or stopping the inflammatory phase. Patients on steroids are often required to stop taking them for a short time before and after surgery.
  - Cancer
  - Major or multiorgan failure.

Extrinsic factors

- *Environment*: This may include the surface on which the patient is lying or sitting; the environment he/she lives in; the support networks available to the patient; social and financial factors. It can also refer to the environment the wound is kept in (see below).
- *Wound dressing*: An inappropriate dressing that maintains an adverse wound environment (e.g. too wet) can cause trauma and/or delayed healing.
- *Clothing and footwear*: These can impact on the healing rates by causing pressure or restriction of blood supply, which means that there is a reduced supply of essential oxygen and nutrients supplied to the wound.
- *Wound site*: Wounds sited over joints (e.g. elbows, knees) will usually take slightly longer to heal than wounds over non-mobile areas.
- *Temperature*: The temperature of the wound bed is of particular importance; ideally a wound ought to be maintained at body temperature (i.e. 36.9°C). If the wound is not dressed with an appropriate (insulating) dressing, the wound bed will cool according to the atmosphere and will result in a reduced blood supply. The body temperature of an individual is also important; the peripheral circulation will be reduced in order to preserve the core temperature, if it is allowed to cool down. This in turn reduces the amount of blood (and therefore oxygen and nutrients) reaching the wound bed.
- *Nutrition*: It is vital that the patient with a wound takes in additional calories in order to increase healing rates, particularly with regard to increased proteins.
- *Wound care skill/technique*: One of the most common reasons for delayed wound healing is the wound care technique of health professionals. This may include the use of inappropriate dressings, causing trauma on removal of the dressing (causing the wound to revert back to the beginning of the healing process); and leaving a dressing in situ for too long, causing saturation and subsequent maceration/excoriation of the wound and peri-wound tissues.

Wound Care at a Glance, Second Edition. Ian Peate and Melanie Stephens.
© 2020 John Wiley & Sons Ltd. Published 2020 by John Wiley & Sons Ltd.
Companion website: http://www.ataglanceseries.com/nursing/woundcare/

The lists discussed in this chapter are not exhaustive, and many unique factors not listed here may apply to the individuals, such as a rare medical condition or a particular lifestyle. In order to ensure that all potential factors relating to any individual are identified, it is vital that a holistic assessment be completed at the onset of the wound, and the patient regularly monitored throughout the healing process for management of all the involved factors. This approach can help ensure that any delay in the wound-healing process is avoided.

13 Nutrition and wound-healing

Figure 13.1 Malnutrition universal screening tool.

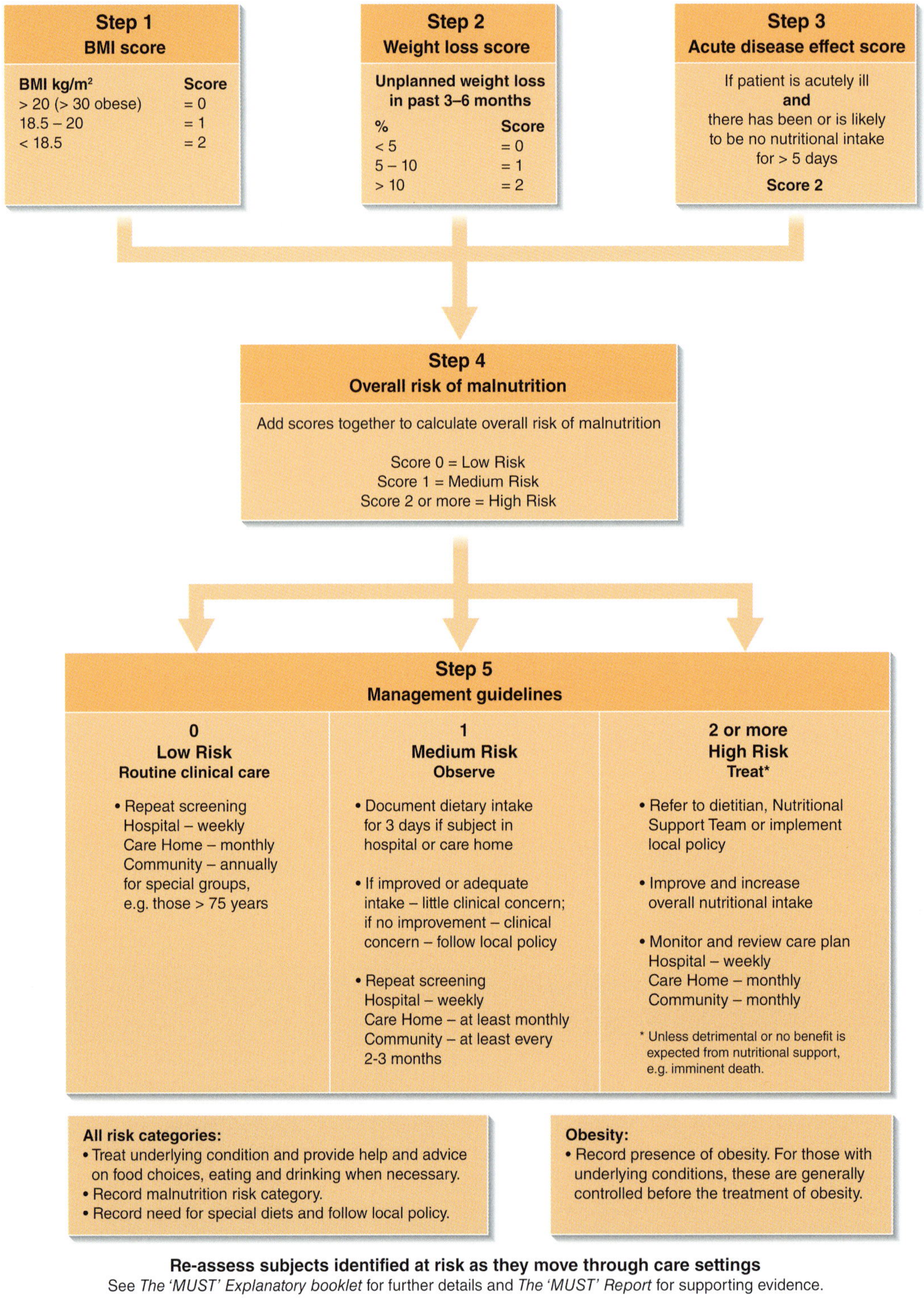

Step 1 — BMI score

BMI kg/m²	Score
> 20 (> 30 obese)	= 0
18.5 – 20	= 1
< 18.5	= 2

Step 2 — Weight loss score

Unplanned weight loss in past 3–6 months

%	Score
< 5	= 0
5 – 10	= 1
> 10	= 2

Step 3 — Acute disease effect score

If patient is acutely ill **and** there has been or is likely to be no nutritional intake for > 5 days
Score 2

Step 4 — Overall risk of malnutrition

Add scores together to calculate overall risk of malnutrition

- Score 0 = Low Risk
- Score 1 = Medium Risk
- Score 2 or more = High Risk

Step 5 — Management guidelines

0 Low Risk — Routine clinical care	1 Medium Risk — Observe	2 or more High Risk — Treat*
• Repeat screening Hospital – weekly Care Home – monthly Community – annually for special groups, e.g. those > 75 years	• Document dietary intake for 3 days if subject in hospital or care home • If improved or adequate intake – little clinical concern; if no improvement – clinical concern – follow local policy • Repeat screening Hospital – weekly Care Home – at least monthly Community – at least every 2-3 months	• Refer to dietitian, Nutritional Support Team or implement local policy • Improve and increase overall nutritional intake • Monitor and review care plan Hospital – weekly Care Home – monthly Community – monthly * Unless detrimental or no benefit is expected from nutritional support, e.g. imminent death.

All risk categories:
- Treat underlying condition and provide help and advice on food choices, eating and drinking when necessary.
- Record malnutrition risk category.
- Record need for special diets and follow local policy.

Obesity:
- Record presence of obesity. For those with underlying conditions, these are generally controlled before the treatment of obesity.

Re-assess subjects identified at risk as they move through care settings
See The 'MUST' Explanatory booklet for further details and The 'MUST' Report for supporting evidence.

Source: The Malnutrition Advisory Group 2004, figure on p. 3. Reproduced with permission of BAPEN.

Good nutrition is essential for wound-healing. A person's nutritional status is a good indicator of his/her ability to heal, as malnutrition can significantly impact on all aspects and phases of wound–healing, leading to delayed healing times. The longer a wound takes to heal the more likely it is to become infected or become complex in nature.

Whilst many patients with a poor nutritional status develop non-complicated wounds that go on to heal without any attention to their diet, many of those with chronic and/or complex wounds and/or conditions require thorough assessment and attention to their nutritional intake to improve healing rates.

A balanced diet consists of nutrients that include protein, carbohydrates, fat, water, vitamins and minerals, as all have a part to play in each of the four phases of wound-healing discussed in earlier chapters. Let us briefly consider each of these nutrients and see how they relate to the healing process.

- *Proteins*: Proteins contain amino acids as their building blocks, which are essential for tissue repair and regeneration. Any deficiency in protein significantly impairs collagen synthesis, granulation tissue formation and angiogenesis, and the maturation phases of wound-healing.
- *Carbohydrates*: Carbohydrates provide the energy in the form of glucose needed to power the repair and regeneration process described previously.
- *Fats*: These are essential in providing an energy source when the carbohydrate sources are depleted. Fat is also required to help with thermoregulation (insulation), and it carries fat-soluble vitamins A, E and K, required for wound-healing.
- *Water*: A dehydrated body leads to a dehydrated wound. A dehydrated wound delays wound-healing, as the migration of granulation tissue across the wound bed depends on a fluid environment, which also aids cell-functioning. Additionally, the wound drains fluid (exudate); and, if the wound surface area is large or the wound is heavily exuding, the patient requires an increased fluid intake over and above the normal requirement of 40–60 mL of water per kilogram of body weight per day, in order to prevent dehydration.
- *Vitamins (A, C, K, B complex, E)*: Vitamin A is essential for healthy skin and epithelial integrity; it promotes granulation, angiogenesis and epithelial tissue formation. Vitamin C is essential for building and maintaining healthy tissues, and it assists in absorbing iron. Vitamin K is essential for blood clotting, thereby allowing the wound to progress through the inflammatory response and beyond. B complex vitamins are a group of eight vitamins that are required for normal immune-functioning and energy metabolism. They aid in white blood cell function and resistance to infection, while improving the tensile strength of the wound. Vitamin E is an antioxidant that helps prevent cellular damage; it decreases the inflammatory phase of wound-healing; it enhances immune function and decreases platelet adhesion.
- *Minerals (zinc, iron, copper, magnesium, calcium, phosphorus)*: All these minerals are important to the wound-healing process. Zinc is an antioxidant vital to cell processes and normal immune function; iron is an essential part of haemoglobin and is required for oxygen transportation to cells to maintain life; copper is required for haemoglobin synthesis and iron absorption and transportation, and increases the strength of collagen fibres; magnesium is essential to all living cells and plays an important role in the transportation of calcium and ions across cell membranes, being important for muscle contraction, nerve impulse conduction and normal cardiac rhythm; calcium is essential for bone formation, remodelling and muscle contraction, fibrin syntheses and blood clotting; and phosphorus is essential for normal metabolism, and is an essential component of many enzyme systems.

Nutritional assessment

A malnourished and/or dehydrated patient is at a greater risk of wound complications, for example, wound dehiscence (primary intention), delayed healing rates, wound infection, sepsis and even death. It is therefore essential that routine assessments and reassessments, including weight measurements, are carried out on a patient with a wound in order to ensure that they are receiving an optimum diet and fluids that are sufficient for wound-healing requirements. A nutritional risk assessment tool must be used in order to assist the practitioner in establishing a risk level, but this must not be used in isolation and the practitioner should not replace this with clinical judgement. Figure 13.1 demonstrates the Malnutrition Universal Screening Tool (MUST) recommended for use by the National Institute for Health and Care Excellence (NICE). This is a simple to use tool that gives an indication of the patient's risk due to malnutrition. A more in-depth assessment and referral is necessary if the patient is deemed to be at risk, and the following clinical characteristics should be noted.

Clinical characteristics of malnutrition

The clinical characteristics of malnutrition and dehydration, that the practitioner must be aware of, are emaciation, obesity, transparent skin, pallor, broken blood vessels in the skin, pale membranes of the eyes, missing teeth or poor dentition, bleeding gums, mouth sores and recent changes in body weight (increase or decrease).

Clinical characteristics of the wound caused by malnutrition

In cases where the patient is poorly nourished, the wound may present stagnant or prolonged healing rates including chronic wounds, repeat ulcerations, pressure ulcer formation, neuropathic ulcer formation and friable tissue on the wound bed (fragile and bleeds easily).

Medical conditions that could lead to malnutrition

There are many medical conditions that make a patient more prone to developing malnutrition, and the practitioner must be extra vigilant in the following cases: diabetes mellitus; intestinal conditions; malabsorption conditions (e.g. coeliac disease); cancer; HIV; obesity, dysphagia and any patient receiving parental nutrition.

14 Incontinence and wounds

Figure 14.1 An incontinence lesion.

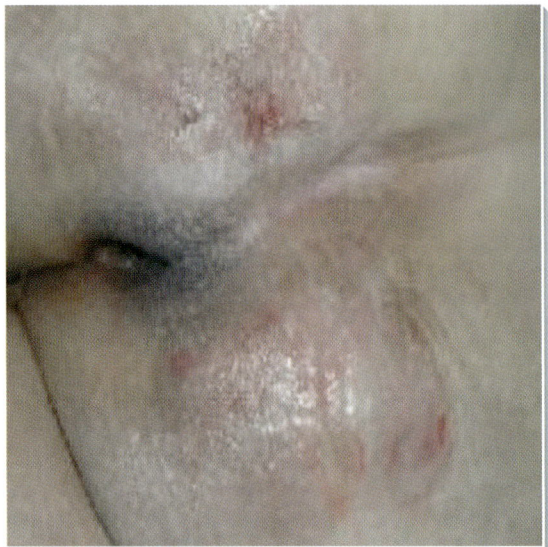

Figure 14.2 Pressure damage exacerbated by moisture lesions.

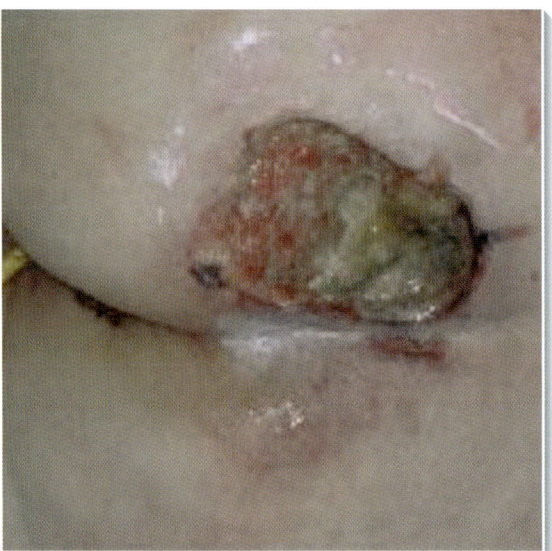

Table 14.1 Features of pressure ulcers and moisture lesions.

Pressure ulcer	Moisture lesion
Usually occurs over a bony prominence, such as over the sacrum, or under anything that applies constant pressure to the skin, for example, under the tight elastic on underwear, or any medical device.	Occurs where there is excess moisture against the skin. The area may be extensive and appears over areas where there are no bones immediately underneath the skin, for example, the buttocks, groins, folds of skin to thighs, abdomen, under breasts. The skin initially looks wet and shiny.
Distinct edges or margins usually round in shape to begin with and confined to the area directly over the bone.	Appears initially as a rash or a tiny graze(s) that is sporadic over the area of moisture. Poorly defined edges may be blotchy.
The onset of pressure damage appears red (when it is Category 1). When pressed, it is non-blanching (i.e. it remains red when pressed; Figure 42.3).	Appears red, and the red area blanches when pressed (i.e. it goes white).
The skin surrounding the ulcer is usually dry.	The skin around the lesions appears 'wet'.
The depth of damage can go deep down to muscle, bones and tendons.	Is usually superficial, although if combined with pressure the damage can go deep as with pressure ulcers. These ulcers are categorised as a combined ulcer. Kissing ulcers and a linear wound to the anal cleft can develop.
Can become infected, although this is unusual with good wound management. Therefore, any infection will be delayed, if at all.	Can usually become infected very quickly due to the presence of bodily fluids and matter that harbours bacterial growth.
Usually hot or lumpy to touch.	Usually cool to touch, unless infected.
The patient complains of pain.	The patient usually complains of a stinging sensation, tingling, burning and itching.

Wound Care at a Glance, Second Edition. Ian Peate and Melanie Stephens.
© 2020 John Wiley & Sons Ltd. Published 2020 by John Wiley & Sons Ltd.
Companion website: http://www.ataglanceseries.com/nursing/woundcare/

What is incontinence?

Incontinence is the unwanted and involuntary leakage of urine or stool. Many people are affected by incontinence across the lifespan and its prevalence increases with age. As the nature of the subject area is considered taboo, fewer than 40% of people seek help with incontinence. When such a problem exists, it can impact on a person's self-esteem, well-being and quality of life. However, the impact on the quality of the skin can be significant unless adequate steps are taken to prevent moisture damage.

The impact of incontinence on the skin

Prolonged contact from the moisture contained within urine and faeces can cause maceration (i.e. overhydration) of the skin and presents as white soggy area of skin; however, due to the acidic nature of bodily fluids, this moisture can also cause excoriation (burning) of the skin, which presents as a red, wet skin (see Figure 14.1).

Once the skin is macerated and/or excoriated, this results in the loss of the protective layer and, therefore, makes the affected area much more vulnerable to damage from bacterial invasion; bacteria multiply in the moisture and the faecal matter and could result in skin infections (cellulitis).

Once maceration and/or excoriation occur, the area also gets much more vulnerable to the effects of pressure and friction, thereby increasing the likelihood and speed at which a pressure ulcer develops, if adequate pressure ulcer prevention and continence care are not provided.

Many people with urinary incontinence restrict their fluid intake believing that this will better control the problem. Unfortunately, this inevitably leads to the dehydrated skin, which is weaker than the well-hydrated skin and, therefore, experiences damage more easily. Additionally, dry skin absorbs moisture from incontinence (and sweating often associated with infection) and becomes macerated or excoriated easier than if it was not dehydrated. Furthermore, dehydration can also lead to urinary tract infections, which in turn result in an exacerbation of urinary incontinence (and sweating) leading to increased risk of moisture damage.

Moisture lesion or a pressure ulcer?

Very often, moisture lesions are mistaken for pressure ulcers, particularly early-onset pressure ulcers (i.e. Category 1 or 2), as they can look very similar in appearance. Figure 14.2 demonstrates a Category 4 pressure ulcer that originated from a moisture lesion. You can see the continued effects of moisture on the skin surrounding the ulcer due to the effects of continued moisture mismanagement. The clinical differences between pressure ulcers and continence lesions are listed in Table 14.1.

Prevention is better than cure

As always, prevention is better than cure. Therefore, to begin with, as far as possible, it is vital to address the causes of the incontinence (or sweating, or both), which include details of the individual's signs and symptoms, a physical examination, review of medications that may increase the risk of incontinence and risk assessment. In any event, it is essential that expert advice is sought from a continence specialist nurse who is able to assess, treat and manage the cause of the incontinence. In the meantime, the following care must be provided and documented in the continence management plan to avoid moisture lesions:

1 Regular routine skin assessment of high-risk areas, observing for inflammation of the surface of the skin with redness, swelling and, in some cases, small blisters containing clear exudate. If there is damage, grade it using the excoriation grading tool.
2 Adopting a structured skin care regimen, which includes the use of a gentle cleansing agent (emulsion, foam or spray) to wash the skin with, patting the skin dry and application of a water-repelling barrier cream/film/spray following each episode of incontinence.
3 Containment of urine and faeces with the use of products that wick moisture away from the skin. This can include the use of urinary sheaths in men, or appropriate fitting, absorbent pads, anal bags and faecal management systems. The continence nurse advises on appropriate products depending on frequency of use and cost.
4 Treatment and management of incontinence through regular toileting, lifestyle changes (reducing caffeine intake, weight loss, adequate hydration, pelvic floor muscle training, bladder training and stopping smoking) and treating of secondary infections.
5 Instigating a repositioning regimen.

15 Vascular disease

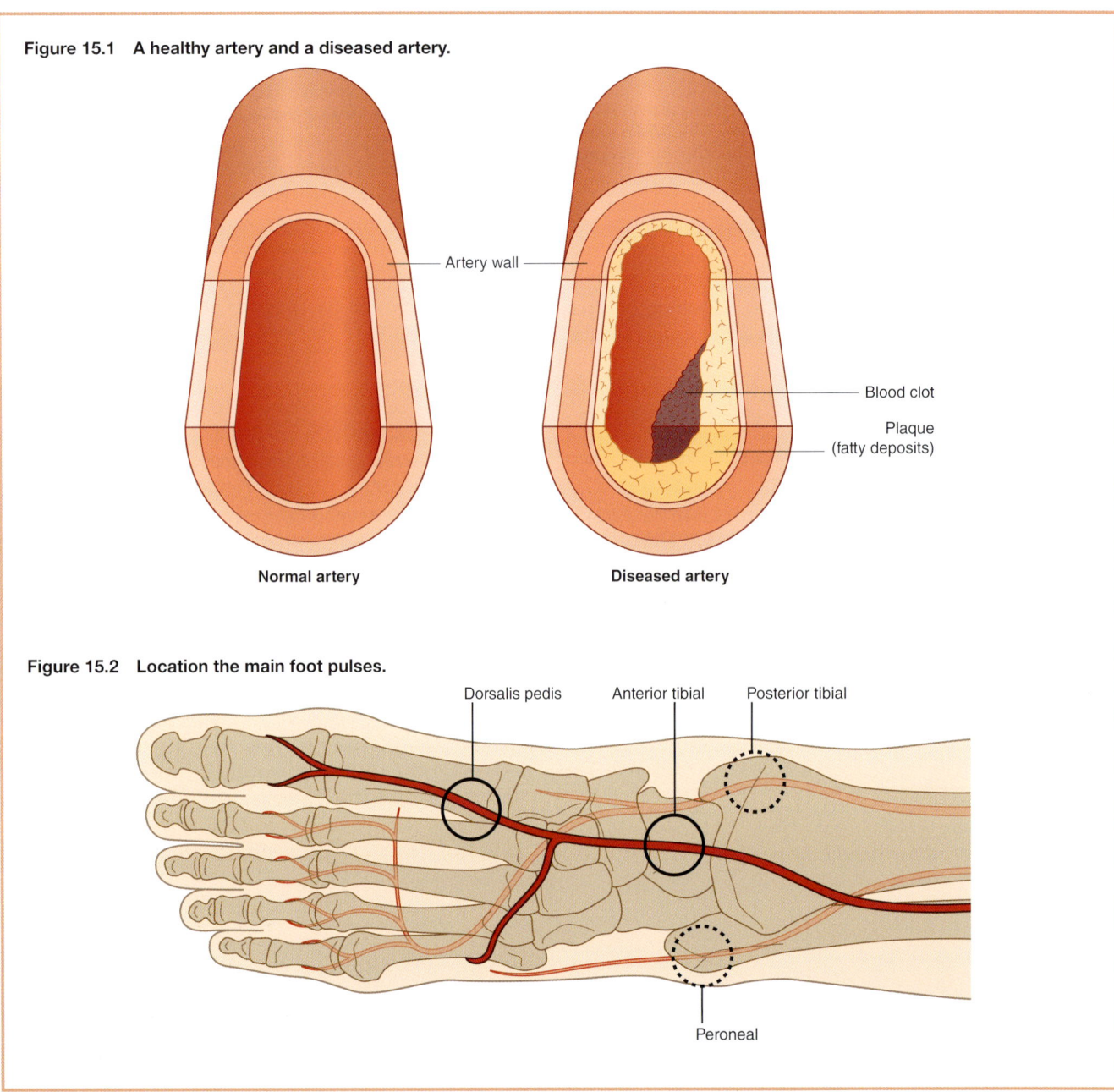

Figure 15.1 A healthy artery and a diseased artery.

Figure 15.2 Location the main foot pulses.

Vascular disease, also known as 'arterial insufficiency', is the lack of adequate arterial blood supply to certain organ(s) or part(s) of the body, which can result in reduced tissue viability or tissue death. The most common type of vascular disease seen in wound care is ulceration to the lower limbs as a result of vascular insufficiency, where limb pain and ulceration may occur due to the lack of blood supply; however, similar issues can develop in the upper limbs.

Lower limb ulcers (arterial ulcers) are the most common type of chronic wound, as many are either very slow to heal or do not heal at all due to varying degrees of reduced or no blood supply to the limb, or parts of the limb. A leg ulcer due to the loss of skin below the knee on the leg takes more than 2 weeks to heal.

Aetiology

Approximately 20% of all lower limb ulceration are due to vascular disease, with the remainder due to venous disease or a combination of venous and arterial disease; around 1% of the population suffers from leg ulceration at some point in their lives. In case of mixed aetiology, it is the more serious arterial disease that must take priority in terms of treatment. Potential common causes of arterial insufficiency include diabetes mellitus (usually microvascular disease), immobility, obesity and rheumatoid arthritis, and can affect any age group.

Arteriosclerosis is a term used for the thickening and hardening of the arterial walls caused by cholesterol deposits that build up on the inside wall of the artery/capillary, gradually narrowing the lumen through which blood travels, thereby reducing the blood supply to the surrounding tissues. It is considered most common in elderly people; other predisposing factors for arteriosclerosis are known to be obesity, hyperglycaemia, hypertension, hypercholesterolemia, smoking and a sedentary lifestyle. Figure 15.1 shows a healthy artery and a diseased artery.

Buerger's disease (i.e. thromboangiitis and thromboangiitis obliterans), which is strongly associated with smoking tobacco, is a condition that develops through recurring inflammation, clotting and vaso-occlusion (narrowing of the medium or large arteries and veins due to the inflammation), caused by carbon in tobacco, thereby leading to a reduced circulation. This condition commonly affects smokers between the ages of 20 and 40 years and is thought to cause an immune response to tobacco in those who are susceptible.

Additional factors that must be considered

Due consideration must be given to the possible presence of generalised vascular disease in patients who have had a cerebrovascular accident (stroke) (by the development of a clot in the brain), those with vascular dementia and cardiovascular disease (e.g. angina and coronary artery disease), those who are given certain drugs, for example, inotropes, that are commonly used in critically ill patients, and those with vascular diseases of vital organs such as the kidneys. Although in these conditions arterial insufficiency is mostly restricted to the specific arteries, there is a possibility that the condition may be widespread affecting other arteries and capillaries. If for example a major artery is occluded due to hypertension (resulting in a stroke), it is possible that the smaller arteries and/or capillaries in the skin could be affected, thus, making the patient more vulnerable to pressure damage or delayed healing of other wound types.

Nursing staff must therefore be extra vigilant in maintaining skin integrity in any patient with any of the aforementioned conditions, as the possibility of them developing wounds anywhere on the body with poor healing rates is too great a risk to ignore. In such cases where a wound does occur, it is essential that the patient is referred for an accurate diagnosis so that the causes of delayed healing can be identified and addressed if possible.

Diagnostic tests for arterial disease

The following are common tests for measuring arterial insufficiency of the extremities:

- *Pulses*: Peripheral pulses must be assessed for all extremity wounds. However, as a decreased blood supply may be affecting the limb (causing a wound), it is possible that the pulse may not be palpated. When checking a pulse by palpation, the rhythm, regularity and strength must be noted. The pulses to be palpated are the femoral, popliteal, dorsalis pedis and posterior tibial pulses of the leg; the brachial and radial pulses of the arm must be palpated in the case of arm ulceration. If pulses are not palpable, they may be heard via Doppler ultrasound. Figure 15.2 shows the location of main foot pulses.
- *Doppler ultrasound*: This involves listening to the sound of the blood pulsating through the arteries using a hand-held transducer. The sound indicates the patency of the artery. A healthy artery has two or three beats that occur as the artery expands and contracts with the flow of blood. These are known as triphasic and biphasic beats. If the artery is compromised, it will usually have only one beat (monophasic) that seems loud and creates a 'gushing' or a 'wind tunnel' sound. This identifies the narrowing, occlusion or hardening (calcification) of the artery.
- *Ankle–brachial pressure index (ABPI)*: This involves non-invasive assessment of the blood pressures in all the four limbs and each of the three arteries of the feet. A calculation is carried out that provides the ratio of the systolic blood pressure of the lower extremities compared to the upper extremities. This establishes an ABPI measurement that indicates the amount of blood that is travelling through each artery, or not, as the case may be. This is discussed in greater detail in Chapters 39 and 40.
- *Capillary refill*: This is a simple test that is a reliable indicator of surface arterial blood flow (i.e. to the skin and tips of digits) and involves pressing on the distal tip of the toe (or finger) for 5 seconds (i.e. emptying surface blood vessels). Capillary refill time is recorded based on the time it takes to refill and regain its original colour. A normal refill time is 3 seconds. A delayed refill time could indicate arterial insufficiency.
- *Rubor of dependency (Buerger's test)*: Briefly, this is a non-invasive test that involves lying the patient supine and noting the colour of the plantar aspect of the foot (the sole). The limb is elevated at varying degrees up, and the colour of the plantar foot is noted. A healthy circulation will not change in colour even at a 60° elevation.

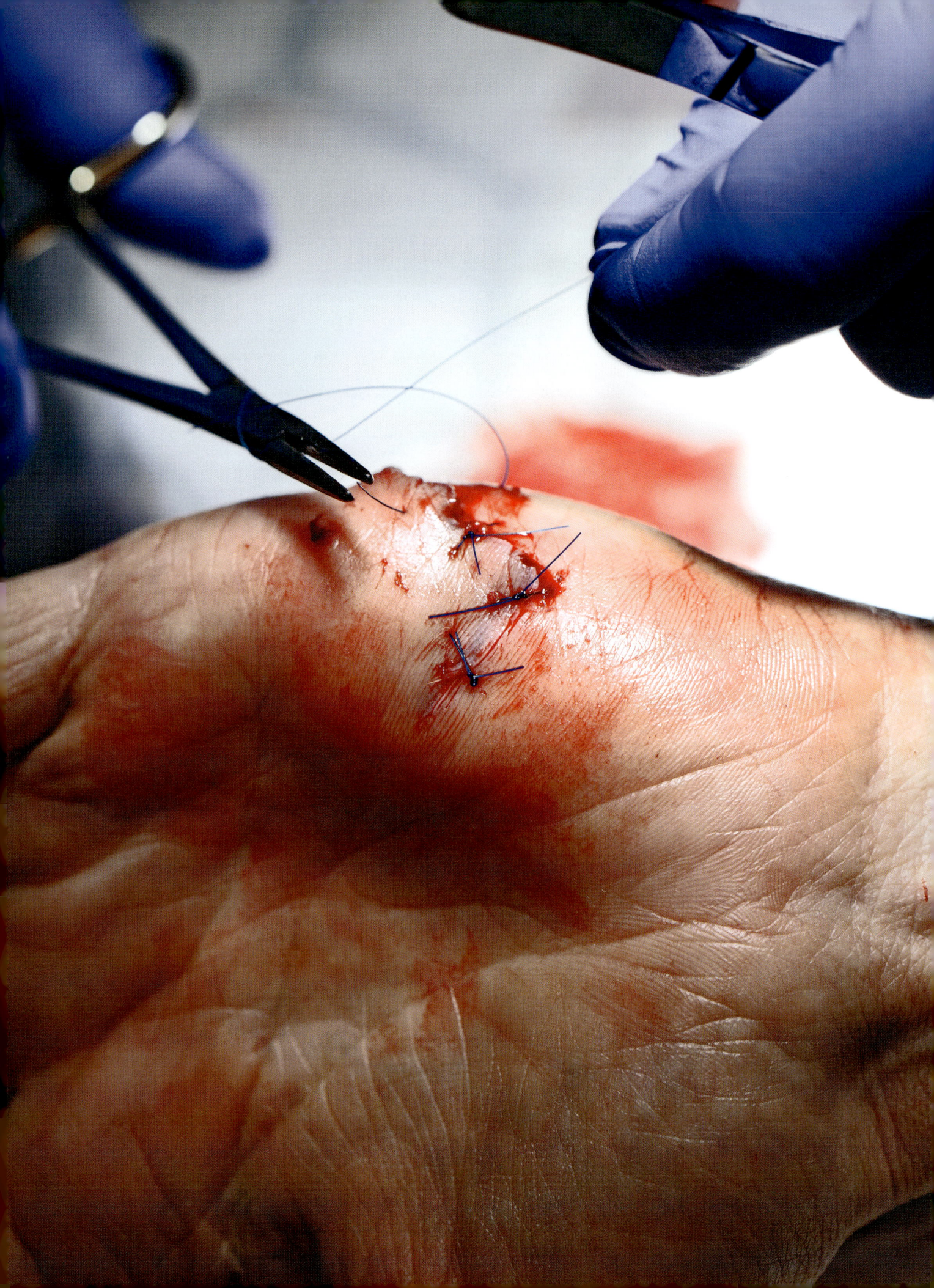

Wound management in practice

Part 4

Chapters

16	Assessment of skin	40
17	Assessment of the patient with a wound	42
18	Classification of wounds	46
19	Legal and ethical aspects of wound care	48
20	Documenting wounds and keeping records	50
21	Evidence-based practice	52
22	Treatment options	54
23	Pain management	56

 Visit the companion website at **www.ataglanceseries.com/nursing/woundcare** to test yourself on these topics.

16 Assessment of skin

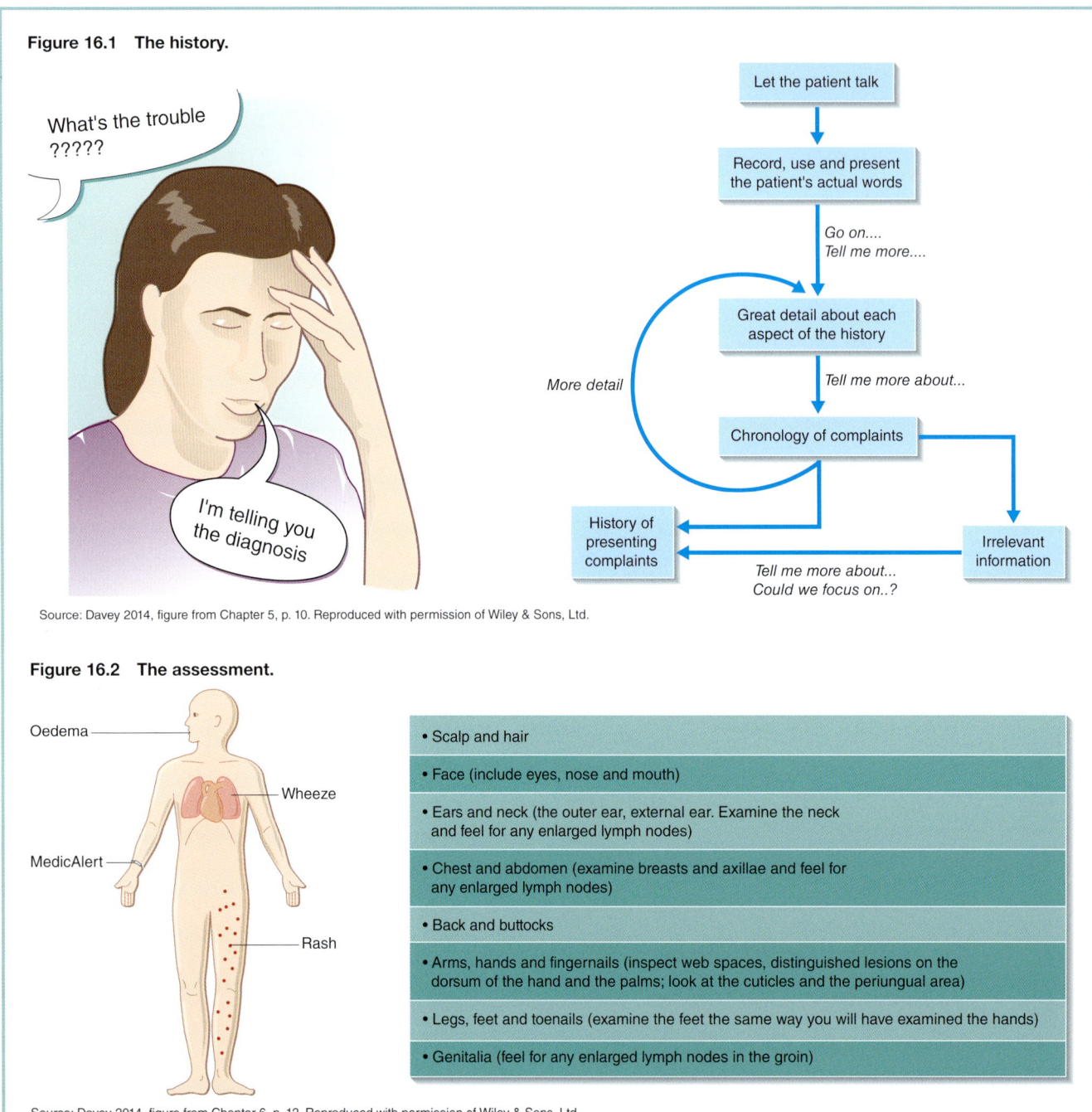

Figure 16.1 The history.

Source: Davey 2014, figure from Chapter 5, p. 10. Reproduced with permission of Wiley & Sons, Ltd.

Figure 16.2 The assessment.

- Scalp and hair
- Face (include eyes, nose and mouth)
- Ears and neck (the outer ear, external ear. Examine the neck and feel for any enlarged lymph nodes)
- Chest and abdomen (examine breasts and axillae and feel for any enlarged lymph nodes)
- Back and buttocks
- Arms, hands and fingernails (inspect web spaces, distinguished lesions on the dorsum of the hand and the palms; look at the cuticles and the periungual area)
- Legs, feet and toenails (examine the feet the same way you will have examined the hands)
- Genitalia (feel for any enlarged lymph nodes in the groin)

Source: Davey 2014, figure from Chapter 6, p. 12. Reproduced with permission of Wiley & Sons, Ltd.

Wound Care at a Glance, Second Edition. Ian Peate and Melanie Stephens.
© 2020 John Wiley & Sons Ltd. Published 2020 by John Wiley & Sons Ltd.
Companion website: http://www.ataglanceseries.com/nursing/woundcare/

The skin is the largest organ of the body and one of the most important. Throughout the lifespan, a person's skin is subjected to a large number of insults; these can be both internal and external and can affect either its structure or function. In a healthy person, the skin is strong and resilient, with the ability to repair itself in response to all but the most severe of insults. However, the skin may be subject to changes that result in making it vulnerable, impaired and dysfunctional. Some of the changes are intrinsic; for example, the effects of skin conditions, ageing or underlying illness, and others are extrinsic and include environmental damage.

Patient history

One of the most important aspects of assessing the skin is to ensure that a detailed history is obtained, eliciting the most salient and important aspects of the patient's story. The amount of time required to take a meaningful history depends upon the person's complaint. Understanding the history should take up most of the time during the consultation. A comprehensive assessment is required.

Diagnosing the underlying cause of a wound is essential. The cause of the wound must be identified; if it is a chronic wound then the underlying factors that may have contributed to or are contributing to the chronicity should be identified so that they can be controlled.

The history provides the practitioner with an essential insight into the key features of the complaint, and this information must be recorded in her or his own words, not masked by medical jargon. The most important skill is to listen and encourage the patient to talk, without interruption. Open questions should be asked so as to elicit as much information as possible; the practitioner may also be required to ask closed questions so as to get to the point or seek clarification. If the patient is not able to provide primary data, then secondary sources of data are required; for example, the relatives, other healthcare professionals or the patient's previous health records should be consulted (Figure 16.1).

The history and summary of the findings must be recorded in the patient's notes. It is also useful to provide the patient with a summary of the findings to ensure correctness.

Past medical history
This is a crucial aspect of the history and should be recorded in detail in chronological order.

Drug history
The determination of what medications the patient is taking and asking them why they are taking them is important, even if it is known what the drug is usually prescribed for. Determine if these medications are prescribed or these are over the counter or herbal remedies. If the person is using topical medications, the practitioner should determine what these are, why the person is using them and how they are using them.

The findings can represent a disease process that is limited exclusively to the skin, or there may be evidence of a systematic disease.

Allergies
The practitioner must determine if the patient has any allergies by questioning. A detailed description of the allergic response to medication or any allergens should be obtained; for example, specific dressings, latex gloves, and so on. The precise nature of the allergy must be identified. Any allergies must be clearly recorded in the person's notes and on drug charts; some people wear MedicAlert-type identifiers, for example, bracelets or pendants.

Smoking
The association between cigarette smoking and delayed wound-healing is well recognised in clinical practice. The patient should be asked if they smoke or have ever smoked. Smoking history, its frequency and its type should also be determined. In a respectful manner, the patient can be reminded about the risks of smoking; this may help them give up smoking.

Alcohol use
Alcohol consumption can increase the risk of infection and interfere with wound closure. Estimating alcohol consumption can help determine if its intake is a potential risk factor.

Physical assessment of the skin

Examination of the skin must go hand in hand with the obtaining of a detailed history (Figure 16.2).

A good light source should be available while examining the skin. The patient should be positioned in a comfortable way during examination; only the relevant areas should be exposed. There are a number of reasons why an assessment or examination of the skin is needed. A number of disease states can be identified on the skin. The findings can represent a disease process that is limited exclusively to the skin, or there may be evidence of a systematic disease. Skin lesions are numerous and present in infinite variations; careful examination and a detailed history help to determine if the findings are confined only to the skin or systemic in nature.

The practitioner may be required to:

- Inspect
- Palpate
- Percuss
- Auscultate.

The examination should include all body surfaces, the skin, nails, hair, as well as the mucous membranes. An entire body examination is not needed if there is a readily recognised lesion (a localised process); however, some vital points may be missed if the practitioner does not look beyond the most apparent pathology or does not listen to the patient carefully about the actual issue. A systematic approach to skin assessment should be adopted and a head to toe approach is recommended. A body map should be used to document the findings.

Assessment tools

There are a variety of tools that can be used to undertake an assessment of the skin. The common tools in use are predictors of risk, risk assessment tools and are related to the assessment and prevention of pressure ulcers. A combination of intrinsic and extrinsic factors can result in the formation of a pressure ulcer. Definitions of pressure ulcers and guidelines concerning assessment and treatment have been provided by the National Pressure Ulcer Advisory Panel and the European Pressure Ulcer Advisory Panel. There are over 40 pressure ulcer risk assessment scales available. Validated scales are used to support clinical judgement, for example, the Waterlow and Braden pressure risk assessment tools. A pressure ulcer assessment tool, called PURPOSE-T tool, has been developed and assesses eight risk factors: mobility; skin; previous pressure ulcer; sensory perception; perfusion (blood flow); nutrition; moisture and diabetes. The Waterlow pressure ulcer risk assessment/prevention policy tool is the most commonly used assessment tool in the UK, and it is also the most easily understood. The tool is intended for use by a number of healthcare professionals and carers. The various skin assessment tools can also be used in conjunction with other risk assessment tools, such as the malnutrition universal screening tool (MUST).

17 Assessment of the patient with a wound

Figure 17.1 A structured wound assessment.

It is the whole of the patient that needs to be assessed when managing wounds – and not simply the 'hole in the patient' – using the following structure.

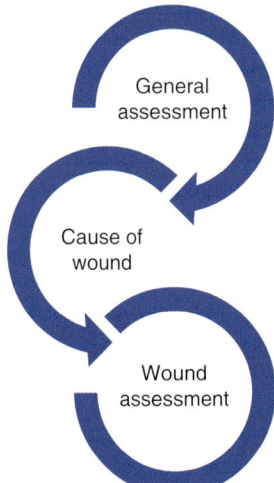

Figure 17.2 The nursing process.

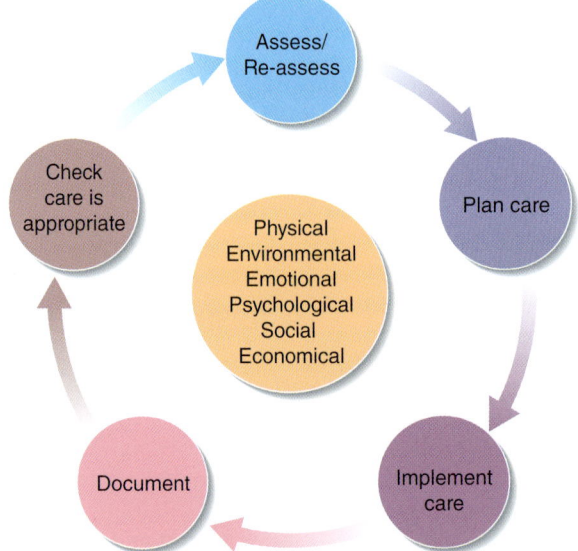

Wound Care at a Glance, Second Edition. Ian Peate and Melanie Stephens.
© 2020 John Wiley & Sons Ltd. Published 2020 by John Wiley & Sons Ltd.
Companion website: http://www.ataglanceseries.com/nursing/woundcare/

As reported in a study analysing 2000 patient records, inconsistencies in the assessment and management of wounds frequently occur with nurses and health care professionals making the common mistake of only looking at and noting the condition of the wound without first considering the patient as a whole, or at all (Guest et al., 2015). The findings reported that 30% of the documented wounds did not have a differential diagnosis, 12% had no diagnosis and only 43% of the wounds had healed within 12 months. The application of dressings and treatments to a wound without a diagnosis and structured wound assessment could potentially mean that the treatment may be contraindicated for a medical condition the patient may have, as the practitioner fails to consider the patient holistically. For example, the practitioner may regularly change the dressing type if the wound-healing is not progressing as it should; this could be because of insufficient eating by the patient to promote healing. The nurse thinks that the wound will eventually heal if she/he selects the 'right' dressing and so continually tries different products on the wound without achieving the desired aim. The nurse fails to consider the patient holistically, and as a result the wound-healing does not progress as it should. In response to this study, in England, improving the assessment of wounds has been specified as a key goal of commissioning. This means that health service providers will have to demonstrate effective wound care delivery and improved healing rates to secure future income while delivering services.

An advanced practitioner or doctor would not prescribe a treatment/drug without first considering the patient holistically, as the failure to do so could cause potential harm or a reaction due to contraindications, and the same principle applies to wound management.

This chapter will therefore consider the importance of assessing the patient holistically rather than simply assessing the wound only. Holistic assessment means that the wound should not be treated separately but in the context of the patient's overall well-being. It will consider the factors that affect healing already discussed in Chapters 10 and 11 and will promote a structured approach to wound assessment to ensure that the patient is considered as a whole rather than simply treating the 'hole' in the patient.

A structured approach to wound assessment

This process is a 360° ongoing cycle of assessment that continually considers anything that could be delaying the wounds progression to healing. It is a process that, when documented, provides evidence to the interprofessional team about the wound's progress and any factors that could be hindering that progress (Figure 17.1).

General health

Firstly, it is important that the practitioner considers the patient's full medical and surgical history, underlying the comorbidities the patient may have and the medications he/she takes to manage the current health condition. For example, the patient may be a diabetic, and it is crucial that blood sugar levels are monitored and maintained within the acceptable levels (i.e. around 5 mmol/L) in order to encourage wound-healing. Many medical conditions are out of a practitioner's control; however, it is vital to manage these appropriately as far as possible. The practitioner must discuss with the patients about any previous treatment they have had for the wound and the achieved outcomes. Several questions must be asked to the patients, such as: Did the wound heal? How often has it reoccurred? Did they experience any sensitivities to dressing products? The practitioner must find out about their current nutritional status and hydration, their age, any allergies and the status of their general health. Some general health issues are unchangeable, such as age, for example. However, other issues can be improved upon, such as the quality of nutrition. It should be remembered that some medical conditions cannot be addressed, and therefore, the wound will not heal; for example, in cases of inoperable peripheral vascular disease, the circulation is so limited that the limb dies due to ischaemia. In such cases, it is vital that the wound environment is maintained to its optimum condition based on the aforementioned assessments.

Lifestyle factors

The practitioner must first stop and consider the environment the patient is being nursed in: Who is providing the nutrition, if anyone? What type of nutrition is that? What type of equipment is the patient being nursed on? Is he/she being repositioned regularly and is this recorded on a chart/care plan or notes? Is the clothing or footwear the patient is wearing ill-fitted? Is the patient still smoking to excess? Is the patient or a relative interfering with the dressings being applied? What is the impact of the wound on the patient's physical, social and emotional well-being, such as sleep, activities of daily life, mobility, altered eating habits, emotions, depression, hobbies, friendships, social isolation, pain and odour? This may take a narrative form, and should also include the level of involvement from both the patient and the practitioner, registering their ability and appropriateness to self-care. Many factors that prevent a wound from healing can be improved upon if identified and given due consideration as part of this process. For example, a patient with the pressure ulcer whose wound is not improving because inadequate pressure redistribution is not being provided will have improved healing rates once frequent position changes are introduced; in other words, the cause of the wound is identified on assessment and adequately addressed (as far as possible) in order to improve healing rates.

Cause of the wound

It is important to assess the cause of the wound. The first few things that must be determined are: Is the wound acute or chronic? How long has it been present? When did it occur? Whether the wound is due to trauma/injury, surgical incision, etc? The wound could be a cause of an underlying disease, such as arterial or venous insufficiency, which would require the practitioner to conduct a Doppler test if necessary. The patient may have diabetes, and may have developed a foot ulcer or a pressure ulcer due to sitting or lying in one position for extended periods of time. If the patient has had more than one wound, each should be assessed individually.

Wound assessment

Once the preceding three steps in the process are completed, it is then essential to assess the wound itself and should be done after cleansing; this includes noting the anatomical site of the wound and the dimensions and depth of the wound. When assessing the dimensions of the wound, it is beneficial to use a tracing, wound map or photography. However, the practitioner must check the local policy and guidance in regard to the informed consent. Also, the practitioner should assess the undermining and tunnelling, as the actual entry site to the wound may be smaller than the damage underneath. Then, the tissue type on the wound bed must be determined and recorded in percentages (e.g. 15% granulation tissue, 60% slough, 25% necrosis, etc.); condition of the wound edges and surrounding skin must be noted (rolled, raised, undermined, epithelialising); levels and type of exudate oozing from the wound should be noticed (none, low, medium, high); signs of maceration or excoriation must be assessed; and signs and symptoms of infection, odour and pain levels, including frequency and aggravating factors for pain, must be recorded.

The preceding findings must then be recorded on a wound chart that lists each of these (see Figure 20.1 in Chapter 20). Reassessments of the wound, along with the patient's general health and lifestyle factors, ought to be carried out at intervals determined appropriate for that wound type, healing rate and health care setting the patient is nursed in. Any referrals on to other members of the interprofessional team – such as tissue viability, leg ulcer, podiatry and vascular services – should be recorded too.

Wound bed preparation

In order to define the treatment goals and optimise wound-healing, it is advised to structure the assessment by using a systematic approach to wound assessment called the TIME framework.

- *T* = Tissue; non-viable or deficient. It is important to differentiate between viable and non-viable tissue, as non-viable tissue will need to be removed in order to promote wound healing, and viable tissue optimised with the appropriate treatment plan.
- *I* = Infection or inflammation. All wounds contain bacteria; however, when wounds are critically colonised or infected, wound-healing is delayed. Swabs, biopsies and treatments using antimicrobials and systemic antibiotics may be considered.
- *M* = Moisture imbalance. A moist wound environment is necessary for wound-healing. One that is too wet or dry requires appropriate treatment in order to assist autolysis, granulation and epithelialisation. Wounds that produce too much exudate may also develop peri-wound breakdown (maceration and excoriation). It is essential that the absorbent dressings and skin protectants are used to prevent leakage and reduce odour.
- *E* = Edge of wound; non-advancing or undermined. It is important to assess the wound edges to observe whether the wound dimensions are advancing and the wound is decreasing in size from epithelial advancement. If the wound edges are not decreasing, then full reassessment is necessary.

Frequency of assessment

It is a minimum expectation that a wound is reassessed (using the preceding process) weekly in the hospital or nursing home setting, and monthly as a minimum in the community setting (e.g. by district nurses) (Figure 17.2). The frequency, however, must be determined by the nurses who are responsible for the patient's wound management and in line with their local policy. If the wound is slow to heal due to age and poor circulation, for example, then fortnightly or monthly reassessments are necessary, provided all the factors influencing the healing rate are recognised and addressed. Until such time, weekly assessments are essential. When a wound is infected, more frequency assessments are necessary in order to monitor the potential systemic infection that renders the patient very unwell, and requiring medical intervention.

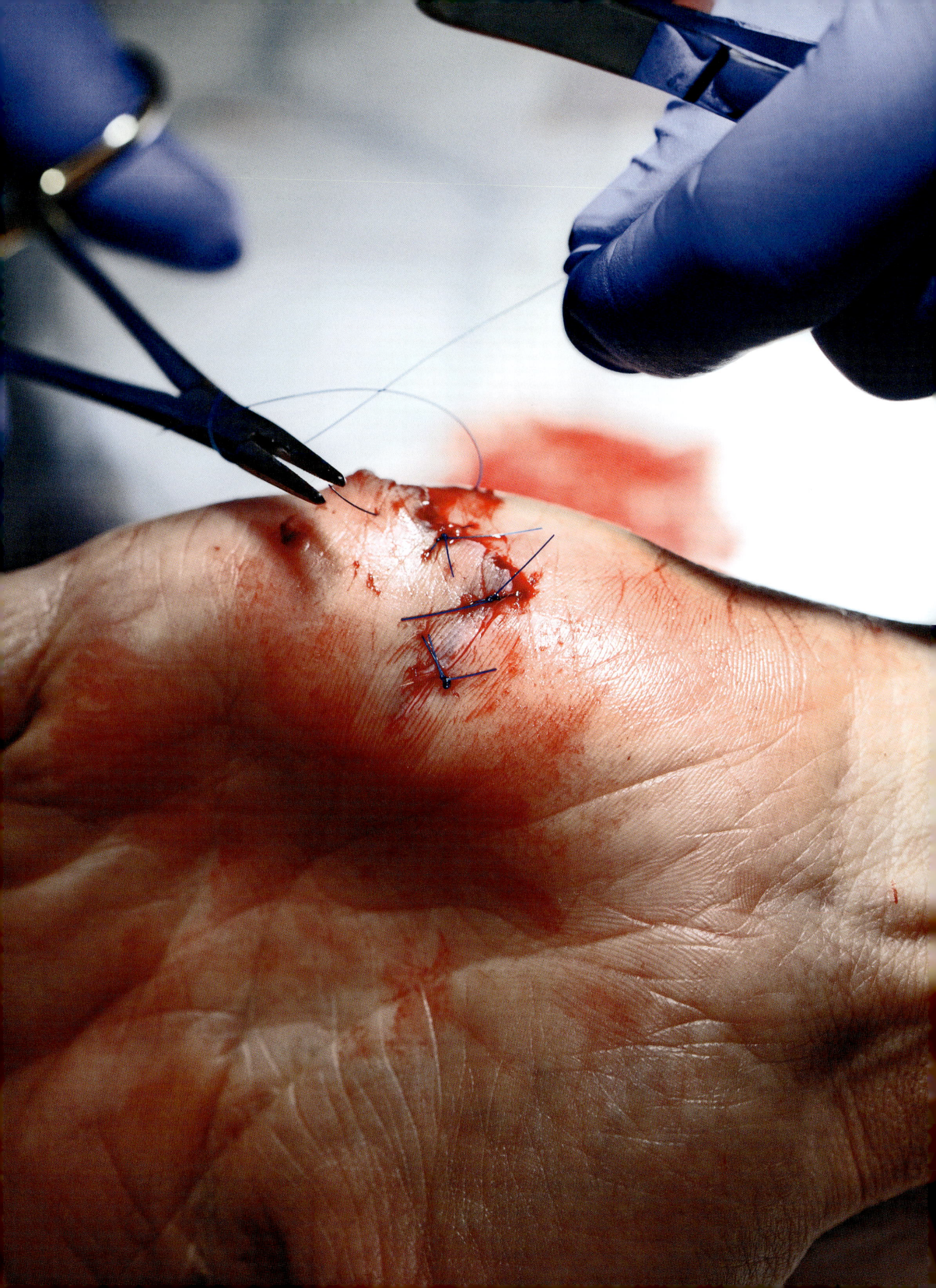

18 Classification of wounds

Figure 18.1 An acute wound (laceration).

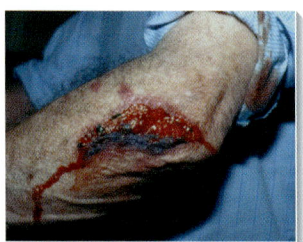

Figure 18.2 A chronic wound (leg ulcer).

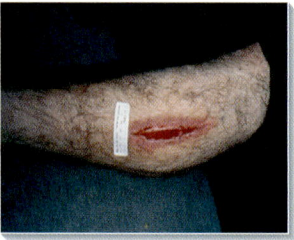

Figure 18.3 A necrotic wound (black).

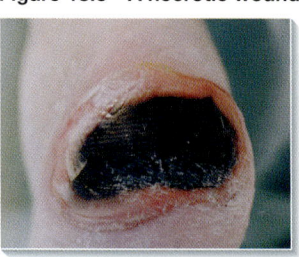

Figure 18.4 A sloughy wound (yellow).

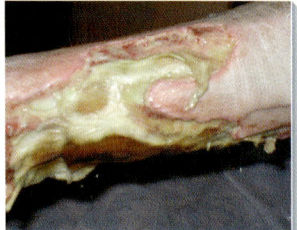

Figure 18.5 An infected wound (green).

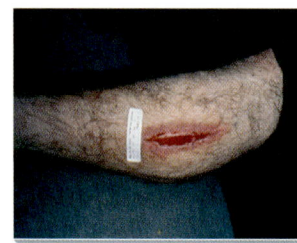

Figure 18.6 A granulating wound (red).

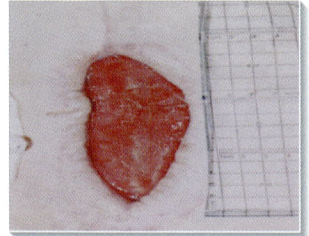

Figure 18.7 An epithelialising wound (pink).

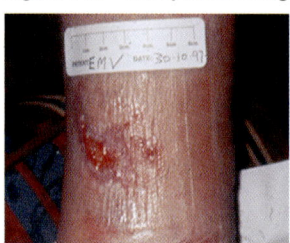

The classification of wounds can be placed into two main categories: acute and chronic. There are two subcategories that identify the phases of the wound-healing process and the tissue type(s) on the wound bed at any given time. The classification of wounds enables nursing staff to accurately assess and plan care for any given wound, taking into consideration the holistic assessment of the patient. It therefore may become evident on assessment of the patient that an acute wound will undoubtedly become chronic due to underlying comorbidities in some cases. There is no definite way to classify wounds; however, the inclusion of the following on a wound assessment form will enable nursing staff to utilise a tool that is neither too simplistic nor complex in order to identify key aspects relating to any given wound, so that appropriate care can be planned.

Acute wounds

An acute wound is induced by trauma or surgery. There are many different causes of trauma, as listed in the following text:

- *Incision*: Sometimes described as a 'cut', this wound is usually induced by a sharp object (e.g. scalpel, knife, shard of glass or a metal sheet) that causes a 'slice' to the skin. There is usually very little tissue loss and the edges are therefore usually very clearly defined. The depth can vary from superficial to deep.
- *Laceration/skin tear* (Figure 18.1): This is usually caused by a blow against a blunt object that causes the skin to 'split'. Often, there is swelling and some tissue loss. It often creates a skin flap that can be very thick or very thin in depth. A skin tear is usually caused by the tearing of the skin by a sharp object, such as a nail, a fingernail, by clothing/belts or rough handling. The frail elderly skin is often subject to this type of trauma. The depth is usually superficial and confined to the skin, but can affect deeper tissues.
- *Burn*: It can be caused by heat (fire), cold (frostbite), chemicals and electricity. It is vital to identify the cause of the burn in order to treat it appropriately. It can vary in depth from superficial to deep.
- *Scald*: It can be caused by hot liquids and steam, and must be quickly cooled. The damage can vary in depth from superficial to deep.
- *Puncture*: A penetrating wound that can be of varying depth caused by pointed objects, such as nails, wooden stakes, pins, needles, teeth (e.g. cat bites), etc. These can appear insignificant due to the small opening on the skin, but underlying structural damage and infection are the risks attached with this wound type. It is possible that a puncture of the skin can occur when a broken bone penetrates the skin.
- *Contusion*: It is a bruise due to the rupture of superficial blood vessels caused by the trauma, without breaking the skin itself. The bruising disperses in around 14 days via the venous and lymphatic drainage, so it requires no topical treatments. The darker the discolouration is, the deeper the damage usually.
- *Friction*: It is the erosion of superficial (and sometimes deeper) tissues caused by the sudden or constant rubbing of the skin against a rougher surface. This type of wound requires healing by secondary intention.
- *Pressure*: This is the tissue death that creates a wound, which is caused by unrelieved and prolonged pressure applied against the skin.
- *Shearing*: This is a closed wound where tissues attached to bone are torn away from the bone due to opposing forces of two types of tissues. The affects are deep seated and can be painful due to inflammation of the bursa tissues at the site of trauma (bursitis). This type of injury is not usually visible to the eye, but makes the patient more vulnerable to rapid onset of pressure damage.

Chronic wounds

A chronic wound is induced by a variety of causes and does not progress through the phases of wound-healing leading to a prolonged or static wound due to underlying causes, usually of a duration longer than 4–6 weeks. The following wound types may become chronic, but any wound from any cause can become chronic due to underlying factors that affect the healing rates:

- Leg ulcers (venous or arterial ulceration) (Figure 18.2)
- Diabetic foot ulceration
- Pressure ulcer
- Some skin conditions (e.g. eczema, psoriasis, blistering, etc.).

Tissue types

The aim of wound management is to prevent the formation of unwanted tissues on the wound bed, while encouraging the growth of granulation and epithelial (healing) tissue in order to repair the wound. The types of tissues are commonly documented in the following colours that can be used as part of documentation, which will be explained in detail in the following chapters. The types of tissues commonly found on a wound bed are:

- *Necrotic tissue* (Figure 18.3) (black): Wet or dry tissue adhered to the wound bed consisting of red blood cells, skin cells, bacteria, varying levels of wound exudate (if moist or wet) and any other debris that may be on the wound, such as dressing fibres or foreign bodies. Necrotic tissue can also consist of gangrene (tissue death). It is important for the nurse to identify what type of necrotic tissue is on the wound, and this will also be discussed later. This is unwanted tissue.
- *Slough* (Figures 18.4 and 18.5) (yellow): Wet or dry tissue consisting of congealed wound exudate, debris, skin cells, bacteria and blood cells. The actual colour of slough varies depending on the ingredients within it. For example, a grey slough has red blood cells, while a yellow slough (Figure 18.4) has many white blood cells within it. A green slough (Figure 18.5) has a bacterium known as pseudomonas within it; however, it must be pointed out that infection is not identified by the colour of slough (discussed later). This is unwanted tissue.
- *Granulation tissue* (Figure 18.6) (red): This is wanted tissue and consists of angiogenesis (new blood vessels) utilised in tissue repair. The aim is to maintain a 'red' granulating wound while preventing the formation of unwanted types of tissues.
- *Epithelial tissue* (Figure 18.7) (pink): This type of tissue demonstrates the covering of skin over the granulation tissue as the wound fills with new tissues. Once the wound is entirely covered with epithelial tissue, the wound is regarded as closed (healed).

19 Legal and ethical aspects of wound care

Wound Care at a Glance, Second Edition. Ian Peate and Melanie Stephens.

Companion website: http://www.ataglanceseries.com/nursing/woundcare/

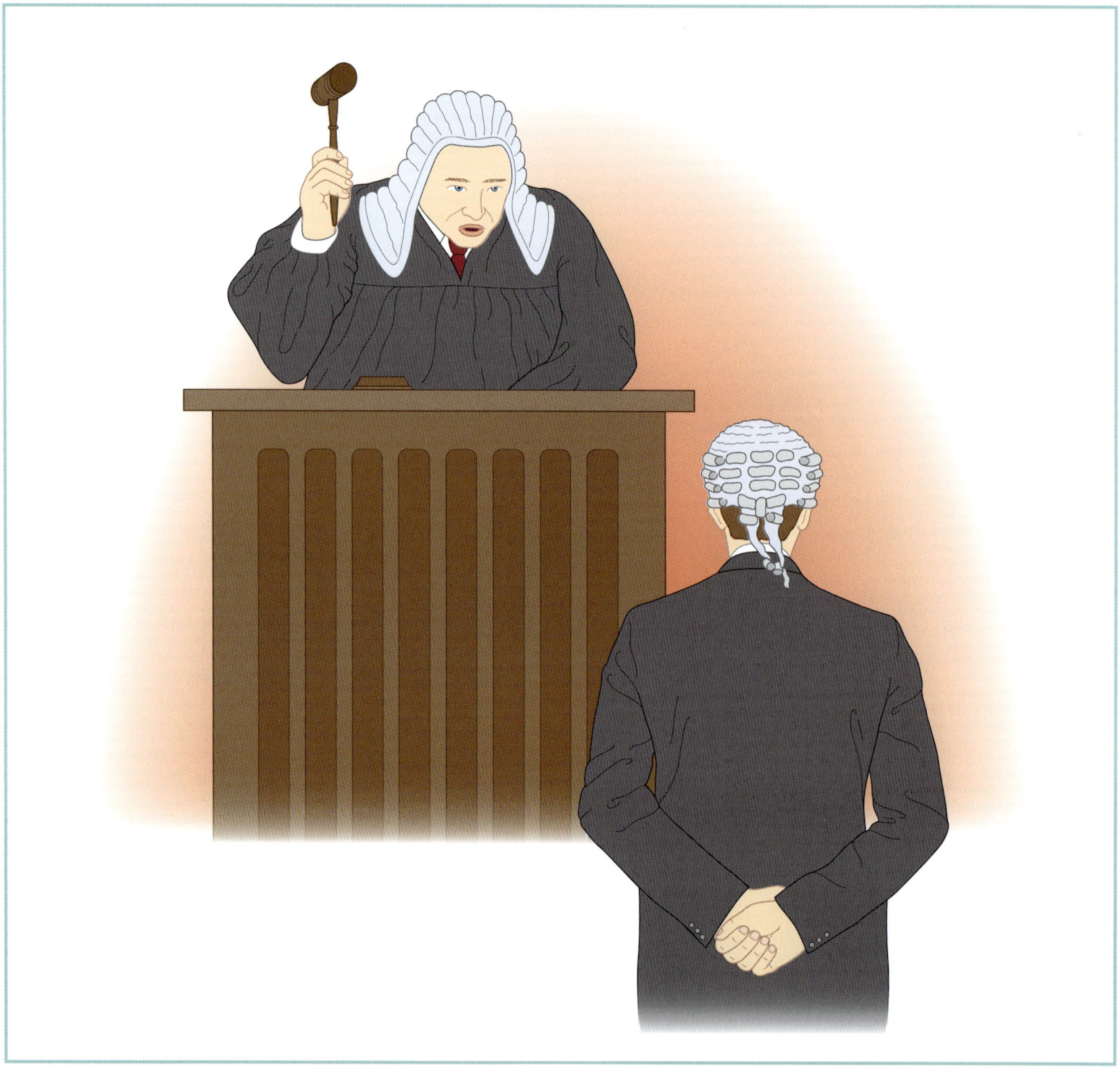

All registered nurses and nursing associates are accountable to the Nursing and Midwifery Council (NMC), to their employer and to the law. All untrained nursing staff are accountable to their employer and to the law. If an untrained nurse works under the supervision of a registered nurse, the registered nurse is held accountable for the untrained nurse's actions. However, all staff are accountable to the patient at any time, and this therefore means that nursing staff must endeavour to adhere to legislation and professional codes of conduct, and must at all times act in the 'best interests' of the patient. With this thought, let us now consider how these professional and legal expectations affect the wound care that is provided to our patients.

Professional standards

According to the NMC, good record-keeping and care-planning is a 'non-negotiable skill that all registered nurses must possess'. They consider it equally important as any other clinical skill required to fulfil the role of a registered nurse. It is commonly regarded that poor standards in documentation is a reflection of the standards of care provided, which would therefore be regarded as equally bad as the standards evidenced in the records.

In October 2018, the NMC released the revised code of conduct that all registered nurses, midwifes and nursing associates must adhere to, titled 'The Code: Professional standards of practice and behaviour for nurses, midwives and nursing associates'. This code states that:

> 'The Code contains the professional standards that registered nurses, midwives and nursing associates must uphold. Nurses, midwives and nursing associates must act in line with the Code, whether they are providing direct care to individuals, groups or communities, or bringing their professional knowledge to bear on nursing and midwifery practice in other roles, such as leadership, education or research. The values and principles set out in the Code can be applied in a range of different practice settings, but they are not negotiable or discretionary'.

The Code comprises of a sequence of statements that when examined together indicate what good practice by nurses, midwives and nursing associates looks like. The four main statements include: *prioritise people, practise effectively, preserve safety* and *promote professionalism and trust*.

> 'You put the interests of people using or needing nursing or midwifery services first. You make their care and safety your main concern and make sure that their dignity is preserved, and their needs are recognised, assessed and responded to. You make sure that those receiving care are treated with respect, that their rights are upheld and that any discriminatory attitudes and behaviours towards those receiving care are challenged.
>
> You assess need and deliver, or advise on treatment or give help (including preventative or rehabilitative care) without too much delay, to the best of your abilities, on the basis of best available evidence. You communicate effectively, keeping clear and accurate records and sharing skills, knowledge and experience where appropriate. You reflect and act on any feedback you receive to improve your practice.
>
> You make sure that patient and public safety is not affected. You work within the limits of your competence, exercising your professional 'duty of candour' and raising concerns immediately whenever you come across situations that put patients or public safety at risk. You take necessary action to deal with any concerns where appropriate.
>
> You uphold the reputation of your profession at all times. You should display a personal commitment to the standards of practice and behaviour set out in the Code. You should be a model of integrity and leadership for others to aspire to. This should lead to trust and confidence in the professions from patients, people receiving care, other health and care professionals and the public'.

In brief, this means that nursing staff, when dealing with patients who have wounds, must first obtain valid consent before treating a patient and taking photographs of wounds; they must respect confidentiality, delegate effectively, use the best evidence available, keep their skills and knowledge up to date, act with integrity, keep clear and accurate records and utilise the expertise of others when it is appropriate. Those records should assist with continuity of care and must be utilised by all members of the interprofessional team. The failure to adhere to these standards could lead to professional sanctions against the nurse, including a 'striking off [the register] order'. It is therefore an expectation that all registered general nurses must be competent in the management of non-complex wounds at the point of entry on the NMC register.

Legal standards

It is vital for registered nurses to ensure that contemporaneous records are kept and that the NMC standards on record-keeping are adhered to at all times. Where documentation is required from untrained staff, it is wise that they too follow the aforementioned principles. At any point in time, those documents and photographs could be seized by the police or by the coroner; they may be requested by the patient and/or the patient's family for use in litigation and therefore the courts, or by the CQC during an inspection of the care setting, all of whom will scrutinise the evidence within those documents and photographs.

Sometimes the staff may be required to account for their previous practice, often several years later, and previous documentation is necessary to do this. Therefore, it is not only in the patient's interests but in the staff's interests as well to maintain high standards of expected documentation at all times. This means that nursing staff are required to produce documentary evidence of the care they have provided to every patient they are responsible for. However, it is commonly stated by members of the nursing/care professions that 'if it isn't written down, then it did not happen', yet despite this common awareness, nursing documentation on the whole is generally poor.

Commonly scrutinised tissue viability issues

Complaints and litigations are on the increase in most care sectors. Common issues are regarding (but not limited to) the prevention and treatment of pressure ulcers; general wound care and wound infections that may have led to sepsis, unnecessary pain and suffering, or even death; suspected abuse or neglect, particularly of elderly people with skin tears, bruising and pressure ulcers; poor skin integrity due to poor nutrition and incontinence.

The standard of the provided care is judged by a court based on the documentary evidence available, including photographs and expert opinion. In reaching this judgement, each nurse involved in the case is measured against the responsible body of registered nurses, skilled in tissue viability, who have not failed to adhere to the standards expected in tissue viability practice at the given time, and to the NMC code of conduct and standards in record-keeping.

If it is found by a court that there was a failure in the duty of care by the nurse or carers (due to lack of documentary evidence to argue otherwise), it is most common that the compensation is paid to the claimant by vicarious liability (insurance policy). The employer may then use its own disciplinary procedures against the nurse, or it may refer the nurse to the NMC. In the most serious of cases, sanctions could include imprisonment of the nurse/carer for wilful neglect, assault and battery, or abuse.

20 Documenting wounds and keeping records

Figure 20.1 NHS Scotland Wound Assessment Chart (reproduced with permission from NHS Scotland).

Wound Assessment Chart
(Use a separate chart for every wound)

Patient ID_____   Wound type_____   Wound site_____

	Initial assessment date	Evaluation date	Evaluation date	Evaluation date	Evaluation date	Evaluation date	Evaluation date
Wound presentation % N – Necrotic (black) G – Granulation (bright red) S – Sloughy (yellow) E – Epithelialisation (pink)							
Exudate colour 1 – Straw colour 2 – Blood-stained 3 – Purulent*							
Level of exudate 4 – None 5 – Minimal (contained within primary dressing) 6 – Moderate (extends to secondary dressing) 7 – High (secondary dressing saturated)							
Other clinical signs of infection 1 – Non-healing/deterioration 5 – Bleeding 2 – Increased exudate 6 – Malodour 3 – Increased pain 7 – Pus 4 – Increased erythema							
Wound traced? Yes or No (please circle)	Y/N	Y/N	Y/N	Y/N	Y/N	Y/N	Y/N
Wound photographed? Yes or No (please circle)	Y/N	Y/N	Y/N	Y/N	Y/N	Y/N	Y/N
Consent for photography obtained? (please circle)	Y/N	Y/N	Y/N	Y/N	Y/N	Y/N	Y/N
Wound dimensions – width, depth, length (cms) EPUAP grade of pressure ulcer 1 – Increasing* 2 – Decreasing 3 – Static* (review treatment)							
Doppler ultrasound assessment carried out? (for leg ulcers) Yes or No	Y/N	Y/N	Y/N	Y/N	Y/N	Y/N	Y/N
Wound odour (a) None (b) Malodorous*							
Wound infection - are there 2 or more clinical signs? Yes or No (circle)	Y/N	Y/N	Y/N	Y/N	Y/N	Y/N	Y/N
Wound swab taken? Yes or No (please circle)	Y/N	Y/N	Y/N	Y/N	Y/N	Y/N	Y/N
Antibiotics prescribed? Yes or No (please circle) (refer to path report)	Y/N	Y/N	Y/N	Y/N	Y/N	Y/N	Y/N
Condition of wound margins, for example, flat, raised, irregular, undermined condition of surrounding skin 1 – Healthy 4 – Oedematous *7 – Dermatitis/eczema 2 – Inflamed *5 – Blistered 3 – Macerated 6 – Ischaemic							
Pain assessment score (see pain assessment documentation)							
Onset of pain caused by? (e.g. walking, dressing change. Please state)							
Pain is relieved by? (e.g. analgesia, elevation. Please state)							
Signature and designation							

Patient's own description of the pain: ....

Additional information: ....

Wound Care at a Glance, Second Edition. Ian Peate and Melanie Stephens.
© 2020 John Wiley & Sons Ltd. Published 2020 by John Wiley & Sons Ltd.
Companion website: http://www.ataglanceseries.com/nursing/woundcare/

In Chapters 17 and 19, we have considered the professional and legal reasons why high documentation standards must be practised at all times and the implications of failing to adhere to these standards. As we have already stated, good documentation is a non-negotiable skill that all nurses must possess according to the NMC, and yet there is an increase in successful litigants who won their case purely because the provision of care was not evidenced in the nursing records. Indeed, this is a common occurrence seen in the most recent project by the Department of Health, known as 'Harm Free Care' and in cases of litigation on pressure ulcers (both discussed in later chapters).

It is therefore important to be clear on the rationale and variety of evidence that can be produced in tissue viability in order to demonstrate the standard of care provided at any given time. But first, we must refresh on the processes involved in producing this documentation.

The nursing process

In the 1970s, Nancy Roper developed the concept of the nursing process using a nursing model that considered the patient holistically by assessing activities of living (ALs), such as eating and drinking, breathing, eliminating and communication. She suggested that when assessing the patient, the nurse must consider social, environmental, physical, economical, spiritual and psychological factors during the process. She argued that, if this is done properly, then no problem, need or risk would go unnoticed by the nurse, who would then be in a position to plan individualised, person-centred care for every health and social care need, problem or risk. The planned care also includes a realistic aim/goal and instruction on how that care is provided. The care must then be implemented, and methods of implementation ought to be evidenced in the patient's documentation. The plan sets a review date where a reassessment of that specific problem, need or risk is carried out in order to ensure that appropriate care continues to be provided. Roper stated that if all ALs are repeated at set dates (e.g. weekly/monthly) to create a continuous 360° cycle of assessment, planning, implement, evaluate (APIE), the patient would be confident that the necessary and appropriate care and/or intervention is provided throughout their entire episode of care in any given care setting.

Tissue viability documentation

Following Roper's principles, let us now consider how good standards in tissue viability documentation can be produced that can provide evidence of acceptable standards of care in accordance with a responsible body of registered nurses.

Assessment

Assessing a wound involves taking note of its anatomical site; dimensions; depth (if a pressure ulcer, this will be by category); tissue type on the wound; levels and type of wound exudate; condition of the surrounding skin (observing for maceration, excoriation, heat on touch and erythema, blistering or any other lesions), pain levels, frequency and aggravating or relieving factors of pain; and whether or not there is a malodour from the wound. This information can be recorded on a wound assessment chart (see Figure 20.1), by photography or by tracing the wound on acetate. All this documentation provides the monitoring that informs all members of the interprofessional team.

Care planning

Once the assessment (or reassessment) is completed, the nurse can establish the aims in order to promote healing. A care plan can then be devised for each identified wound that instructs others on the management. The plan must include a minimum identification of the site of the wound; the aim of the care plan; the type of dressing(s) to be applied to the wound; the frequency of dressing changes and a date when the wound must be reassessed. The plan must be clear and concise and should allow others to deliver the care that has been planned.

Implementing care

Wound care must be carried out using either an aseptic technique (utilising sterile dressings) or a clean technique (utilising warm tap water and dressings). Once the care is delivered, this must be documented in the evaluation chart, the content of which should reflect the directions of the care plan.

Checking the appropriateness of the care plan

Whilst in acute settings, care home or care home with nursing facilities, the wound dressing must be observed at least once on every shift for signs of wound exudate strike-through (i.e. the staining on the outer dressing). Whether or not there is any strike-through, the findings must then be recorded on the care plan evaluation document. Once the dressing shows evidence of strike-through, the dressing requires changing in order to avoid saturation and increased risk of a wound infection. On removal of the dressing, the nurse must check the wound in order to establish whether or not the wound shows clinical changes, and that the care plan remains appropriate if the findings are unchanged.

Making adaptations to the care plan

This may include increasing the frequency of dressing changes, or a different dressing choice to manage the exudate levels more appropriately. Rationale for any adaptations to the care plan must be documented in the care plan evaluation.

Reassessment

In the event the clinical findings are noted to have changed (as detailed in the section titled 'Checking the Appropriateness of the Care Plan') when redressing the wound (e.g. increased exudate levels, signs of infection, increased pain and deterioration in the wound), the nurse must reassess the wound once again (as stated in the section titled 'Assessment'); all findings must be recorded in the evaluation chart, and the care plan either amended or rewritten accordingly in order to reflect the changing requirements and aims of wound healing.

In the event that no clinical changes are noted on daily checks or on dressing changes, then reassessment must be completed at intervals established by either clinical judgement or by weekly/fortnightly/monthly timeframes, as stated by the 2010 regulated activities.

21 Evidence-based practice

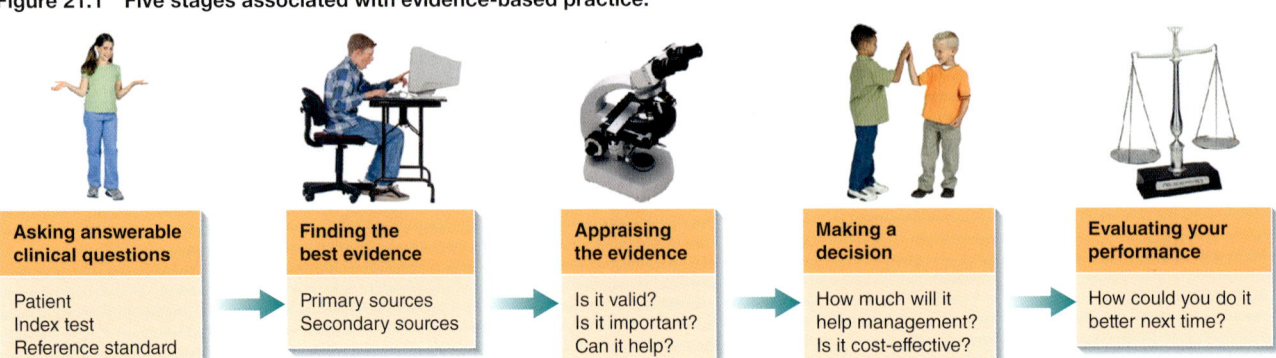

Figure 21.1 Five stages associated with evidence-based practice.

Asking answerable clinical questions
Patient
Index test
Reference standard
Target disorder

Finding the best evidence
Primary sources
Secondary sources

Appraising the evidence
Is it valid?
Is it important?
Can it help?

Making a decision
How much will it help management?
Is it cost-effective?

Evaluating your performance
How could you do it better next time?

Source: Thompson and Van den Bruel 2011, figure on p. x of Introduction. Reproduced with permission of Wiley & Sons, Ltd.

Table 21.1 Hierarchy of evidence.

Level	Description of evidence	Strength
I	Systematic review or meta-analysis of all relevant randomised controlled trials (RCTs), or evidence-based clinical practice guidelines based on systematic reviews of RCTs	Strongest
II	Evidence from at least one well-designed RCT	
III	Evidence from well-designed controlled trials without randomisation	
IV	Evidence from well-designed case-control and cohort studies	
V	Systematic reviews of descriptive and qualitative studies	
VI	A single descriptive or qualitative study	
VII	The opinion of authorities and/or reports of expert committees	Weakest

Wound Care at a Glance, Second Edition. Ian Peate and Melanie Stephens.
© 2020 John Wiley & Sons Ltd. Published 2020 by John Wiley & Sons Ltd.
Companion website: http://www.ataglanceseries.com/nursing/woundcare/

Because of the assortment of wound aetiologies along with their associated comorbidities, a variety of healthcare professionals from all healthcare settings, with each one having a different knowledge base related to wound healing, deliver wound care. There is a need to standardise care and encourage optimal practice in wound management, with the key aim of improving patient outcomes. National guidelines for wound management are being developed. The background and justification for these guidelines provide the health professional with the rationale for their development, associated with information relating to prevalence, potential patient outcomes and resource issues, but they must be derived from an evidence base.

Practising evidence-based wound care will encourage practitioners to integrate valid and useful evidence with clinical expertise and each patient's unique features, enabling the practitioner to apply evidence to the treatment of patients.

Evidence-based wound care

Healthcare practice with a focus on wound care demands the highest level of evidence. Evidence-based wound management is the combination of best research evidence with clinical expertise and patient values. When a practitioner engages in evidence-based practice, they combine their expertise, acknowledging the patient's condition, using the best scientific evidence and listening to the patient's preferences.

Wound care has often been taught through case examples and what was deemed the best clinical practice. There are many elements of wound care that are, and in some instances continue to be, based on hearsay, custom and practice, with little thought being given to why things are done in a specific way.

With the increased importance of providing an evidence base to practice, there is now a requirement to move away from indiscriminate clinical practice, experiential learning, associated with outmoded, unjustified opinions, to learning that has an evidence base. The evidence available extends from expert opinion to randomised clinical trials.

Healthcare practitioners (in line with clinical governance requirements) must strive to provide the safest and best quality care they can. Evidence-based wound care practice requires thought along with a questioning approach to patient care. Evidence-based wound care is required because of the increasingly complex nature of healthcare and healthcare decisions; it is essential that services and treatments be based on the best evidence of what works and what does not work, and they should be able to demonstrate adherence to the various codes of professional conduct.

Five stages of evidence-based practice

Evidence-based practice can be divided into a number of stages. These are the five stages associated with evidence-based practice (Figure 21.1).

Asking answerable clinical questions

The first step is recognising that there is a need for new information. This information need is likely to be vague, and as such it is required to be converted into an answerable question in order to facilitate an efficient search for the answer. Precise answers can only be provided when a precise question is posed. The question should be carefully framed, helping to determine what type of evidence is to be found. It is not unusual for a number of questions to emerge at the same time; and it is not possible to answer all of them at once. Failure to ask a focused and precise clinical question can be a major threat to evidence-based practice.

Acquiring and finding the evidence

Choosing the right evidence is of central importance. There are various sources of evidence, and it can be hard to know where to begin. The main sources of evidence often come from more experienced colleagues and textbooks; however, there are problems with these sources of information. How can you be sure that the information that colleagues provide is reliable? When using evidence from textbooks, the opinions expressed may be out of date before the book is even published, or incompatible with current best evidence. A number of groups have established levels or hierarchies of evidence, usually based upon scientific merit in an empirical model. When examining evidence, it is helpful to consider the hierarchy of evidence (Table 21.1).

Assessing the evidence

The evidence must be critically appraised to establish its validity and potential usefulness. The main questions to ask when appraising the evidence are:

- Can the evidence be trusted?
- What does the evidence mean?
- Does this answer the question?
- Is it relevant to practice?

There are different appraisal and interpreting skills that can be used, depending on the kind of evidence being considered.

Arriving at a decision, acting on evidence

Once it is decided that the evidence is of sound quality, another decision is needed to be made whether the evidence should be incorporated into clinical practice – change. Consideration of both the benefits and risks of implementing the change, as well as the benefits and risks of excluding any alternatives should be undertaken. These decisions should be made in collaboration with the multidisciplinary team, managers and patients where appropriate. Resistance to change should be given serious consideration, as this can be a challenge. Involving all key stakeholders (colleagues, patients, carers, budget-holders and commissioners) can help ensure that the change is implemented as well as sustained.

Evaluation and reflection of performance

Evaluation and reflection are essential to determine whether the action(s) taken have achieved the desired results. This is a fundamental aspect of healthcare practice.

Evidence-based practice is a continuous, cyclical process. Once each stage of the process is worked through, it is likely that new questions will arise and will need to be answered. Evidence-based wound care should focus on employing a questioning approach to your practice. This should not be seen as a 'one-off' activity. It is a continuous process that can help you provide safe and high-quality care to patients. An evidence-based approach can assist practitioners in their own professional development, as they question and seek evidence-based solutions.

22 Treatment options

Figure 22.1 Closure by primary intention.

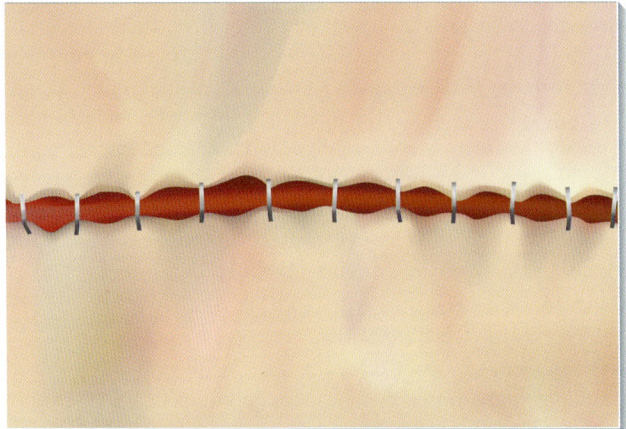

Source: P. Vong. Reproduced with permission of P. Vong.

Figure 22.2 Closure by secondary intention.

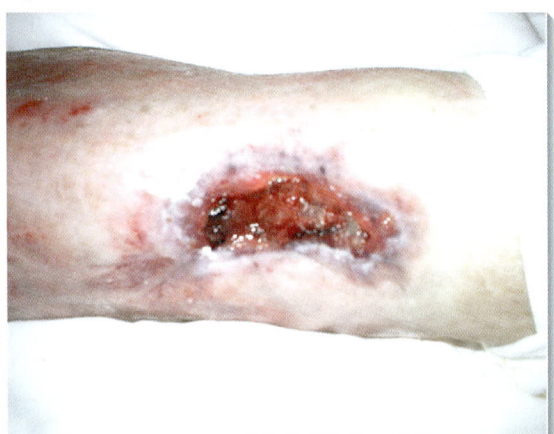

Figure 22.3 Larval therapy.

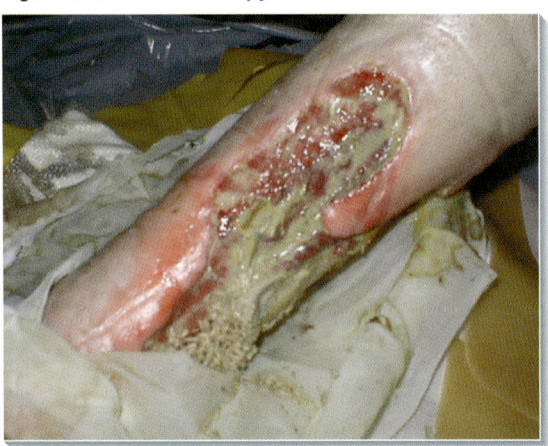

Figure 22.4 Topical negative pressure system, for example, VAC negative pressure wound therapy.

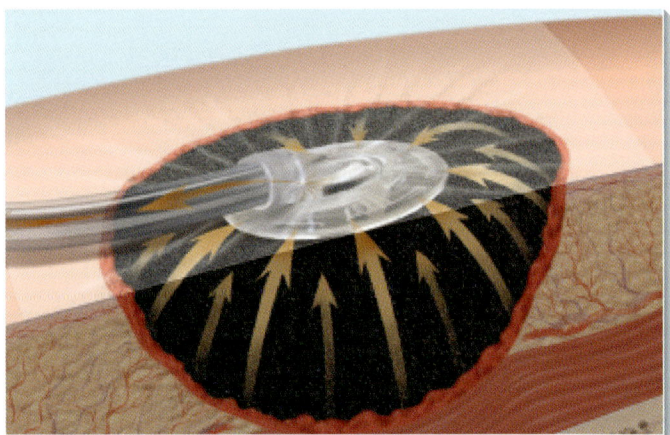

Source: KCI. Used with permission. Courtesy of KCI.

Wound Care at a Glance, Second Edition. Ian Peate and Melanie Stephens.
© 2020 John Wiley & Sons Ltd. Published 2020 by John Wiley & Sons Ltd.
Companion website: http://www.ataglanceseries.com/nursing/woundcare/

Wound closure

When faced with a normal wound or a chronic wound, the assessing nurse must consider treatment options that address the clinical findings of the wound and to promote healing rates. The choices made depend on assessment of the wound, as well as on the patient. So, when a wound first occurs, the initial treatment option that must be considered is wound closure. There are two common types of closures.

- *Primary intention* (Figure 22.1): It is the closure of a wound by the use of mechanical aids, such as sutures, staples, strips, glue or a combination of these, to hold the edges of the wound together. It can only be used on wounds where there is little or no tissue loss and where the margins of the wound can be held together by these aids without undue tension on them. If the tension on the aids is too much, the wound dehisces (i.e. pulls apart), and it has a greater surface area, requiring healing by the secondary intention.
- *Secondary (tertiary) intention*: It is done when a wound is left 'open' and allowed to heal by contraction, without the use of mechanical aids other than dressings, for a number of reasons: too much tissue loss to pull and hold the edges of the wound together; the wound has dehisced due to swelling, infection or too much tissue loss; or the primary intention is contraindicated due to a high risk of infection, particularly common with abscesses and animal bites, for example.

In either case, the wound progresses through the phases of wound healing discussed in the earlier chapters. The difference is that the healing can be visualised in wounds that heal by secondary intention, whereas with primary intention, the healing rate occurs underneath the line of closure. In the meantime, a third method is also used in some cases, described in the following text.

- *Delayed primary intention*: This is used where a wound is initially allowed to heal by secondary intention and later closed by primary intention. The delay allows for reduction in swelling that could cause a wound to dehisce (e.g. a surgical wound), or it allows for treatment of infection in cases of abscesses or infected wounds (e.g. animal bites and boils that have been lanced). If an infected wound is closed by primary intention, for example, this 'seals' in the bacteria that multiply under the closure line, causing the wound to dehisce. Many experts argue that this type of closure should not be used in any event, as once the wound surface area is colonised with bacteria, this will be sealed in when the wound is eventually closed. This type of closure must therefore be carefully considered.

Treatment options for secondary intention healing

If primary intention closure is not suitable, or if part of a wound closed by this method requires secondary intention closure, the next consideration for the nurse is to select the most appropriate treatment for the wound. The treatment options available depend on the findings on wound and holistic patient assessment, and on the aims of the wound at the given time. Let us now consider common options used in the UK.

- *Surgical debridement* (Figure 22.2): This is the mechanical removal of dead and devitalised tissues on the wound bed (e.g. necrosis, slough and gangrene) or the removal of infected tissues. It is carried out by a surgeon or advanced practitioner under the influence of an anaesthetic (local or general) and may involve the removal of healthy tissues, so that the wound may bleed. It is often carried out on wounds that require rapid cleansing due to infection or the risk of infection, particularly on the most vulnerable patients. However, the risks of surgery must be weighed against the benefits of alternative methods, such as autolytic debridement.
- *Sharp debridement*: It is a method used by doctors, or nurses trained in this method, to mechanically remove unwanted tissues from a wound (e.g. slough or necrosis). It can be done at the bedside or in a clinic, does not require an anaesthetic and entails the removal of dead tissues only. It does not involve cutting into healthy tissue, so the wound should not bleed. Owing to this limitation, it is not always possible to remove all of the unwanted tissues, and a combination of this and other methods may be required to fully debride the wound of unwanted tissues.
- *Larval therapy* (Figure 22.3): This is a method of tissue removal (slough, necrosis or gangrene) by the use of maggots. The larvae excrete an enzyme that liquefies the unwanted tissues. The larvae then drink this liquid, thereby cleansing the wound bed. While drinking this liquid, the larvae also swallow the bacteria present within the liquid, and the bacteria are then eradicated in the gut of the larvae. One treatment of larvae can remove a moderate amount of slough/necrosis; however, several treatments may be required before the wound is fully cleansed.
- *Autolytic debridement*: This is a method of removal of dead and devitalised tissues on the wound bed (e.g. slough or necrosis) by the use of dressing products that create the optimum environment, whereby the unwanted tissues are prevented in the first instance, or get liquefied and absorbed into the dressing in the second, until the wound is fully cleansed of unwanted tissues. In other words, the action of maggots is almost mimicked, but without using an enzyme. Instead, body's own moisture is of advantage that exudes onto the wound, provided a moist environment is maintained on the wound. That moisture liquefies the unwanted tissues, whilst the dressing absorbs the excess liquid away. In cases where a wound is dry, or if the patient is dehydrated, hydrating products can be used to achieve the moist environment in order to kick-start the debridement process.
- *Topical negative pressure/negative pressure wound therapy* (Figure 22.4): This is a method of wound healing that can only be used once the wound is free from dead and devitalised tissues, and usually follows any of the above methods of debridement. Negative pressure is applied to the wound bed, which then promotes an increase in the blood supply to the wound bed. This increases the rate of angiogenesis, and, therefore, the growth of granulation tissue. It removes excess exudate, thereby maintaining a moist wound-healing environment. As it removes the exudate, it maintains minimal levels of bacteria on the wound bed, thereby reducing the risk of wound infection whilst it is in operation. Healing rates with this method are usually quicker than with traditional methods of healing. Topical negative pressure is also known as vacuum-assisted closure (VAC).

Generic wound products with over 3000 types of wound dressings are available; it can easily become stressful thinking about which one should be used to manage the patient's wound. However, there are basic properties of the eight main categories of wound dressings, which will be discussed in more detail in Chapter 27. The prescription costs of advanced wound and antimicrobial dressings in the community in England were nearly £106 million in 2016–2017; and, due to the lack of robust clinical or cost-effective evidence, most UK healthcare organisations have a wound care formulary. A formulary is an accessible framework to assist in appropriate dressing selection for nurses and other healthcare practitioners. The framework provides details of each available organisation-approved dressing for use in wound care. This includes a list of uses, contraindications, dressing characteristics, precautions, sizes, cost and examples of an 'appropriate' wound for treatment by a particular dressing. A formulary is used alongside regular mandatory training to develop awareness about wound care, encouraging evidence-based clinical decision-making and practice and promoting accountability.

23 Pain management

Box 23.1 Comprehensive pain assessment summarised by the NOPQRST mnemonic.

Number of painful sites

Origin of pain (what causes your pain?)

Palliative/provocative factors (what relieves the pain or what makes it worse?)

Quality of pain (what words would you use to describe the pain?)

Region/radiation of pain (does the pain travel to other parts of your body?)

Severity of pain (on a scale of 0 to 10, how severe is it?)

Temporal aspect of the pain (does the pain get worse at night? Is it constant or intermittent?)

Figure 23.1 Visual analogue scales for pain assessment.

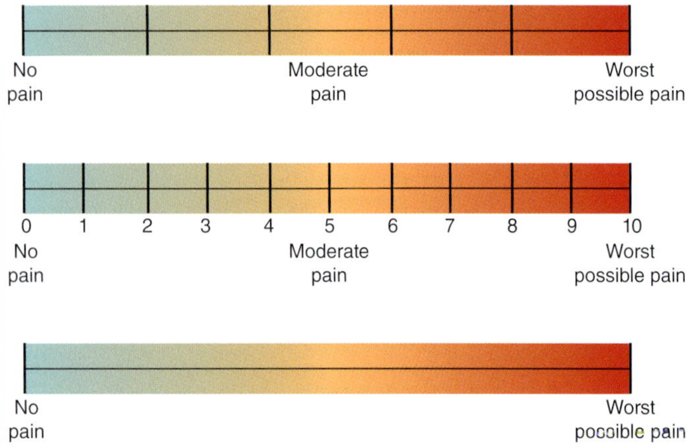

Figure 23.2 The WHO analgesic pain relief ladder, adapted from the World Health Organization.

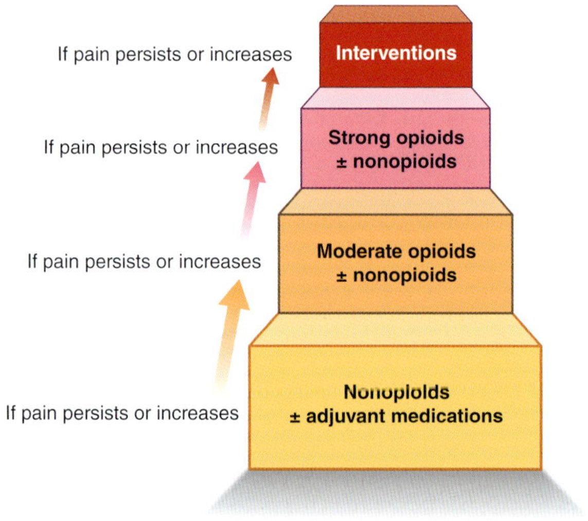

Wound Care at a Glance, Second Edition. Ian Peate and Melanie Stephens.
© 2020 John Wiley & Sons Ltd. Published 2020 by John Wiley & Sons Ltd.
Companion website: http://www.ataglanceseries.com/nursing/woundcare/

Pain – a holistic approach

Pain, just as it is with most issues in wound care, can be complicated. The pain associated with a specific tissue injury that resolves in a time frame related to the degree of injury is *acute pain*. *Chronic pain* is less well-defined and can be related to tissue damage (nociceptive pain) or nerve damage (neuropathic pain), or there may be a combination of the two. When infection is present, this provides another pain dimension and wound care interventions. The pain that patients experience can also be unrelated to the wound, for example, rheumatoid pain, but related to wound care, specifically when positioning a patient for an intervention and the provision of analgesia. The pain experienced when a dressing is being changed is not therefore always limited to the wound itself. Along with the physical components of pain, there are also psychological and emotional factors exacerbating how a patient perceives pain. The various wound aetiologies bring with them different challenges related to pain and its consequences; for example, in diabetic neuropathy, there is an absence of protective pain sensations, which can lead to significant tissue damage; the acute pain experienced by burns results in severe pain. Other challenges have to be faced in palliative wound care when this is related to advanced disease, as the person nears the end of life. Pain management is a significant element of wound care, bringing with it a number of issues and challenges that require a sound evidence base and a multidisciplinary approach.

It is only in the last decade that there has been more appreciation of the role of pain in the life experience of those with wounds. Those patients with wounds such as leg ulceration are said to experience significantly greater bodily pain than the normal population. This phenomenon is not simply a consequence of an older population; it is more a feature of the wound in association with an underlying abnormal pain mechanism.

Wound-related pain

Wound-related pain can be described as an unpleasant symptom or experience directly related to open skin; it can be background pain, that is, chronic or persistent, that may be experienced most of the time. This is compared to an acute incident/procedure-related pain that can arise as a result of routine dressing changes or operative procedures, such as biopsy or debridement. Pain is a subjective sensation that is best described by patients as a result of their personal experience.

There are several individual factors that can influence the pain experience, including anxiety and pain expectation. Exacerbation of pain occurs when other local wound care factors are present, including dressing change, wound cleansing, debridement, presence of infection, bacterial damage and inappropriate choice of dressing.

Unrelenting chronic background wound-related pain can have a significant negative impact on the person's abilities to perform the activities of living, impacting on health and well-being. Experiencing wound-related pain could be seen as one of the most devastating aspects of living with a chronic wound.

To minimise pain, various strategies (pharmacological and non-pharmacological) must be considered at the time of wound care–related procedures, including dressing change. A detailed assessment of pain is required, so that plans may be put in place to anticipate pain-relieving needs; an evaluation on interventions must be carried out to determine effectiveness.

Pain assessment

It is an established fact that pain improves significantly with effective treatment, which promotes healing. Yet, there are some instances where practitioners may be unconcerned or unwilling to accept the degree of suffering of patients from pain related to wounds. Assessing pain associated with wounds is a skill that must be underpinned by a sound knowledge base.

Wound-related pain can change over time, requiring frequent reassessment. Dressing change has been identified as the most painful aspect of wound care, as well as pain at rest between dressing changes and during the performance of daily activities. Pain assessment can help to distinguish the background pain from the pain that is procedure provoked. Ongoing assessment of pain can help to determine the temporal pain pattern for selecting and planning appropriate pain interventions, to assess the efficacy of pain treatments/interventions, to consider factors that may enhance or exacerbate wound-related pain and to identify barriers that can affect pain management.

Comprehensive pain assessment can be summarised by the mnemonic NOPQRST (Box 23.1). There is a selection of visual analogue scales available that can help the practitioner in assessing pain (Figure 23.1). It must be remembered that pain is not a one-dimensional experience; there are multiple factors that impact on pain, and other important information is needed to ensure that a holistic and thorough assessment has been done. Providing patients with a list of words can help them describe the pain they are experiencing.

Pain management

Choosing the right treatment depends on the outcome of the assessment. The practitioner should consider local treatment for pain, as this brings with it fewer side effects. There are strategies that include the use of wound products that are moist, analgesia impregnated dressings and the application of topical analgesia.

There may also be a need to consider systemic treatment, and this choice should not be solely based on size or type of wound; it must be based on the outcome of the assessment and need. Adherence to pain management protocols can guide treatment, and the World Health Organization pain relief ladder produced in 1986 can provide a framework to apply (Figure 23.2). Since its introduction, further pharmacological and interventional approaches have become available. Adjunct therapies, such as muscle relaxants and steroids, can be used to enhance the effectiveness of analgesia. In some specific types of pain, such as neuropathic pain, anticonvulsants or tricyclic antidepressants can be used.

The emotional needs of the patient must be given consideration, as pain associated with the wound can trigger psychological distress. Psychological distress can cause explicit manifestations of stress. Stress impacts on the ability of the body to heal; in such cases, referral to a psychotherapist may be needed.

The key components of pain management associated with wounds include improving access to appropriate products, developing the knowledge base and undertaking a detailed holistic assessment of the person and their pain.

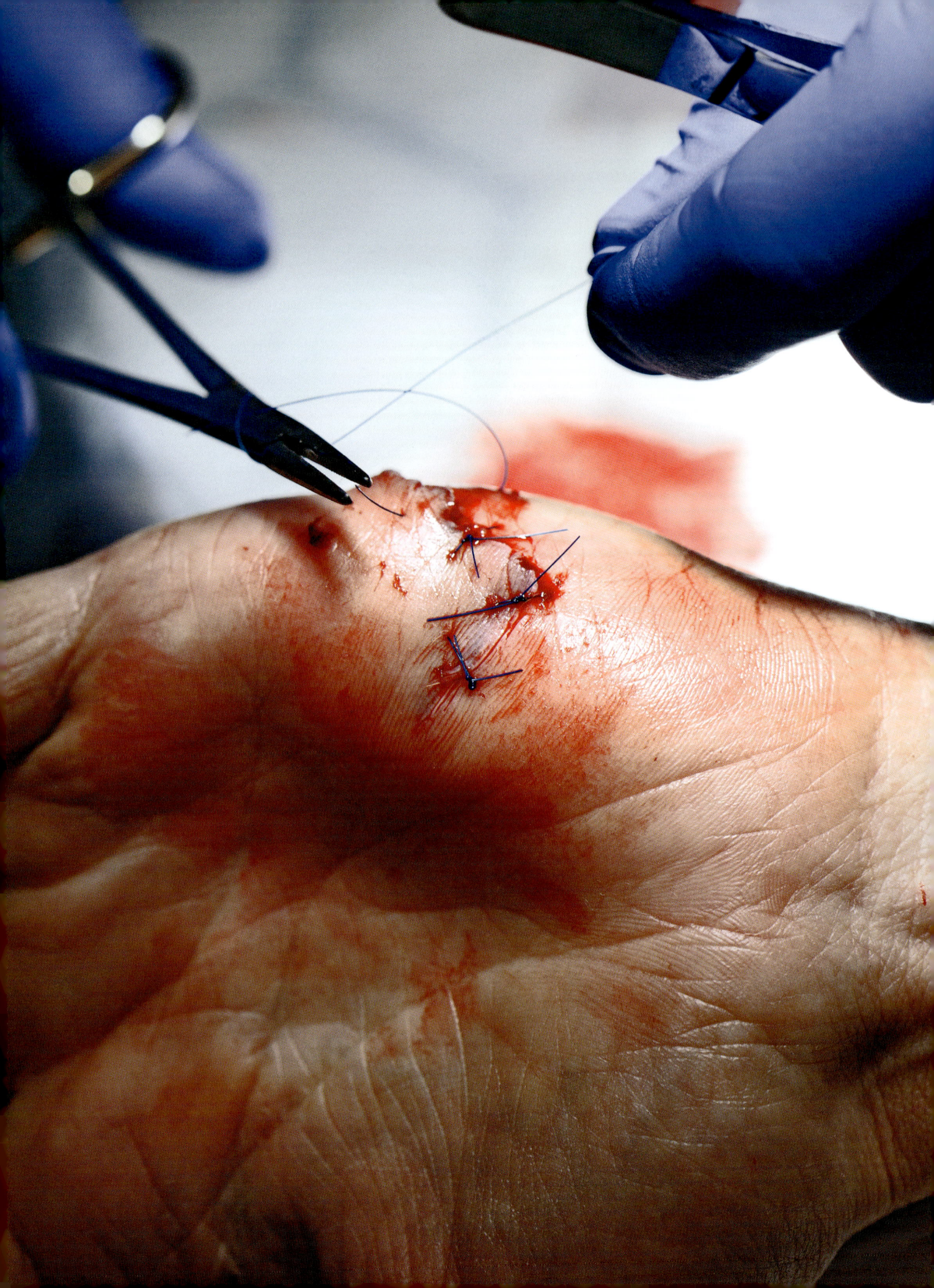

Dressing selection

Part 5

Chapters

24	Principles of wound management I	60
25	Principles of wound management II	61
26	Managing wound exudate: moist wound healing, hydration and maceration	62
27	Generic wound products: mode of action	64
28	Choosing a wound care product	68
29	Use of topical antimicrobials and antibiotics	70
30	Application of lotions, creams, emollients and ointments	74
31	Advanced technologies	76

 Visit the companion website at **www.ataglanceseries.com/nursing/woundcare** to test yourself on these topics.

24 Principles of wound management I

Applying principles

Before a dressing or a treatment can be applied to a wound, it is crucial that a full assessment be carried out (i.e. holistic and wound assessments). Any underlying causes of the wound must be addressed as far as possible and any factors that affect wound-healing rates must be dealt with in the best possible manner. This must be maintained on an ongoing basis. One classic error that tissue viability nurses frequently remark on is that nursing staff continually change the dressing or treatment, believing that this will encourage the wound to heal, but fail to address the underlying causes or factors that hinder healing; for example, with a pressure ulcer, nursing staff frequently fail to provide adequate pressure relief and/or fail to ensure a patient is eating sufficient nutrients that will promote healing. The nurses just change the dressing type when the wound fails to heal. It must, therefore, be clear that it is the patient's own body that heals the wound and not the dressing, which simply provides an environment that promotes the healing rates if used appropriately; otherwise, the wound-healing rates get delayed.

The following principles must then be applied to the management of the wound.

Wound irrigation: This is not always necessary; in the event of a traumatic wound, whereby a wound may be contaminated with debris and bacteria, it may be essential to irrigate the wound thoroughly to get rid the wound of contaminants. Care must be taken in the event of underlying bone fractures or exposed tendons and the patient may need to be transferred to a minor injuries or accident and emergency department for specialised care and treatment.

In most wound cases, however, simple tap water irrigation gets rid the wound of more contaminants and bacteria as compared to the wound that is treated with the non-sterile solution. In cases of a new surgical wound, if there is an underlying fracture, or if the patient's general health is compromised, it is advisable to use sterile saline to irrigate the wound.

The frequency of wound irrigation depends on its clinical findings; for example, if there is any loose debris that can be removed by irrigation. If the wound is infected, or if there are high levels of wound exudate that make it more prone to infection, then it is advisable to thoroughly irrigate the wound to reduce (but not eliminate) the bacterial levels, which helps return the pH levels of the wound to come within normal range over time. Once the exudate levels reduce to a 'moist' level, provided there is no loose debris on the wound, then a weekly irrigation can be carried out to maintain control over the bacterial levels that inevitably multiply over time if irrigation is not done at all. Although irrigation does not remove all bacteria, it reduces the number of bacteria on the wound bed. Without such irrigation, bacteria numbers simply increase until the wound becomes critically colonised and healing is unable to progress.

It must, however, be kept in mind that unnecessary irrigation simply delay wound healing, as brand-new vulnerable granulation or epithelial cells can be easily damaged or washed away. Therefore, a fine balance must be achieved.

When irrigating a wound, it is vital that gauze swabs are not used and that the irrigating fluid is poured over the wound instead. Using gauze simply causes trauma and pain on wound contact and simply spreads the bacteria around the wound without removal.

Wound swabs: It is general practice for a wound swab to be used when clinical signs of infection are present in order to assist in identifying the causative bacterium. There is little benefit in using a wound swab when the wound is progressing towards healing, as the bacteria living on the wound are clearly insufficient to hinder the healing rates. With good irrigation at timely intervals and the use of appropriate dressings, the wound healing should continue to progress, provided all other holistic factors influencing the healing rates are also addressed.

In the event that a wound swab is obtained, the results depend on what part of the wound the swab has made contact with; as bacteria live in colonies, it is possible that the causative bacteria may not make contact with the swab, so inappropriate antibiotics are often prescribed. Similarly, any wound can be contaminated or colonised with bacteria, so any swab used on even a healthy, non-infected wound can grow microbes. Therefore, care must be taken to avoid unnecessary use of antibiotics that could lead to bacterial resistance, placing the patient at risk of prolonged healing rates.

Aseptic technique: The principles of aseptic technique must be applied when dealing with any wound; the use of sterile gloves is not necessary for older wounds, but gloves must be changed after removal of the old dressing, and again after wound irrigation in order to apply the new dressing. In cases where there are underlying bone fractures, a new surgical wound or if the patient is immune-compromised, it is advisable to use sterile gloves throughout, changing them at the steps already stated.

In all circumstances, a sterile dressing must be applied to the wound from an unopened, undamaged product wrapper. Any unused dressings must be disposed of and should not be kept for future use.

Pain control: Prior to commencing with dressing changes or wound treatments, it is vital to assess the patient's pain levels using an appropriate pain tool; analgesia must then be given as necessary, allowing sufficient time for this to take effect before wound care is commenced. Reassessment of pain should be carried out following dressing change, and this is discussed in greater detail in another chapter.

Maintaining the preceding principles, let us now look at the application of dressings in the following chapter.

Principles of wound management II

As stated in previous chapters, the aim of wound management is to achieve a 'moist' wound-healing environment, with the exception of the necrotic, ischaemic wound, which must be kept dry in order to minimise the risk of developing gas gangrene. Apart from this, the only other exception to moist wound healing is with the overgranulating tissues. If the wound is too wet, it requires absorbent dressings; if it is too dry, the wound needs rehydrating, either by insulating the wound so the body can donate moisture or by adding moisture using hydrating products, such as hydrogels or hydrocolloids. In any event, once a wound reaches a 'moist' level, it is not necessary to add moisture with hydrating products.

Care must be taken when using hydrating products, and the holistic health of the patient must be considered, as donating moisture too quickly will increase the speed of bacterial growth, thereby placing the patient at increased risk of infection. In such cases, it is safer to treat a wound 'conservatively' by insulating the wound with an appropriate dressing that allows the body to donate the necessary moisture spontaneously. While this is a safer option, it is a much slower method to debride the debris from a wound than if hydrating products were used; therefore, risks versus benefits must be considered. Additionally, the patient's oral intake of fluids must be encouraged, so that the dehydrated patient's wound remains dry. The risks versus benefits of hydrating a wound must be analysed, aiming to achieve and maintain a 'moist' wound balance.

Typical care plan to manage wound moisture levels

This should detail the site of the wound and the aim of the care plan; as a minimum, it should describe the necessary steps required, such as when to irrigate a wound, include the dressing type(s), frequency of dressing changes and when the wound ought to be reassessed.

A crucial aspect of maintaining a moist wound environment is the frequency of dressing changes; if a dressing becomes saturated, the moisture that is produced by the wound has nowhere to go, macerating the surrounding skin. If a wound is very wet, it may require several dressing changes in a day and cause maceration an excoriation of the peri-wound skin; if a wound is very dry, it may not need changing very often. The nurse must, therefore, observe the dressing for signs of exudate strike-through. It is not advisable to leave a dressing in situ for longer than 7 days, even if there is no strike-through visible.

A typical wound management care plan is provided in the following text that would be suitable for most wounds. Please be aware that all deeper wounds or cavity/sinus wounds require filling with a suitable dressing (not a hydrogel). If a hydrofibre or an alginate is placed directly on any wound bed, it creates a moist environment only if it is covered with a modern insulating dressing; otherwise, it dehydrates and adheres to the wound bed, as the moisture is evaporated through a non-insulating dressing.

Wound management care plan

1. After removing the dressing, irrigate the wound bed, which helps to reduce the risk of trauma whilst removing debris, microbes and excess exudate.
2. Gently pat dry the surrounding skin; do not touch the wound bed.
3. Apply a primary dressing, depending on the clinical findings and depth of the wound, as follows:
   (a) If the wound is moist or wet, use a hydrofibre, alginate, lipido-colloid dressing or foam dressing directly on the wound bed;
   (b) If the wound is infected, use an antimicrobial dressing on the wound bed until the infection resolves;
   (c) If the wound is dry, consider using a hydrating product (only after the risks versus benefits have been considered and found to be appropriate).
4. Apply a moisture barrier to the peri-wound skin; allow it to dry.
5. Cover the wound with an appropriate secondary dressing, as follows:
   (a) If the wound is wet, use an absorbent foam dressing;
   (b) If the wound is moist, use an absorbent foam dressing, film dressing or a hydrocolloid, based on assessment of risk versus benefits;
   (c) If the wound is dry and the patient is fit and healthy with no ischaemia of the wound, a hydrating product can be used;
   (d) If the wound is dry and the risks of using hydrating products outweigh the benefits, the debridement/rehydrating process can be stimulated by moistening about 10% of the alginate or hydrofibre dressing before applying it to the wound, then cover it with either a foam (for a longer wear time) or a film dressing.
6. Observe the dressing for signs of exudate strike-through.
7. Change the dressing immediately after the exudate strike-through appears and repeat the preceding process. This will avoid maceration of the peri-wound skin and granulation tissue and will maintain a moist environment.
8. Record each dressing change on the care plan evaluation, noting any concerns/changes in the wound. If necessary, reassess the wound.
9. Reassess the wound weekly, fortnightly or monthly (depending on the care setting and speed of healing), and record the findings on the wound assessment chart (Figure 20.1).
10. *Remember*: Risks versus Benefits = Moisture Balance.

Wound Care at a Glance, Second Edition. Ian Peate and Melanie Stephens.
© 2020 John Wiley & Sons Ltd. Published 2020 by John Wiley & Sons Ltd.
Companion website: http://www.ataglanceseries.com/nursing/woundcare/

26 Managing wound exudate: moist wound healing, hydration and maceration

Figure 26.1 A moist/damp environment.

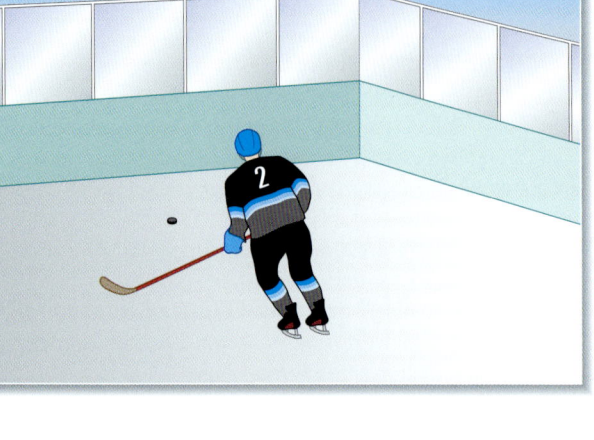

Figure 26.2 A moist/damp wound environment.

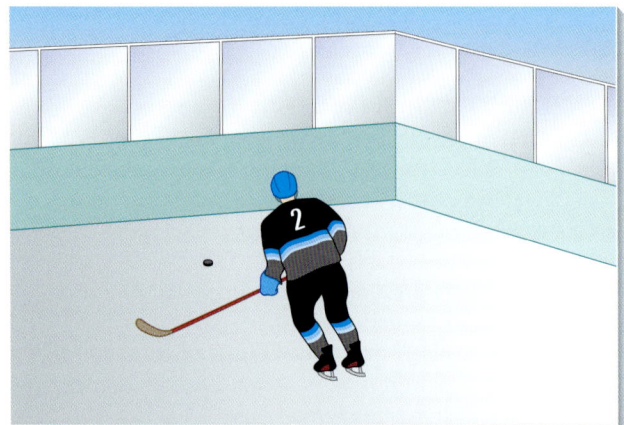

Figure 26.3 A dry environment.

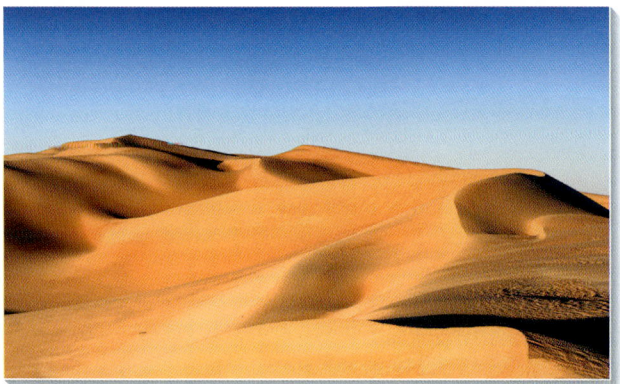

Source: iStock © hadynyah.

Figure 26.4 A dry wound environment.

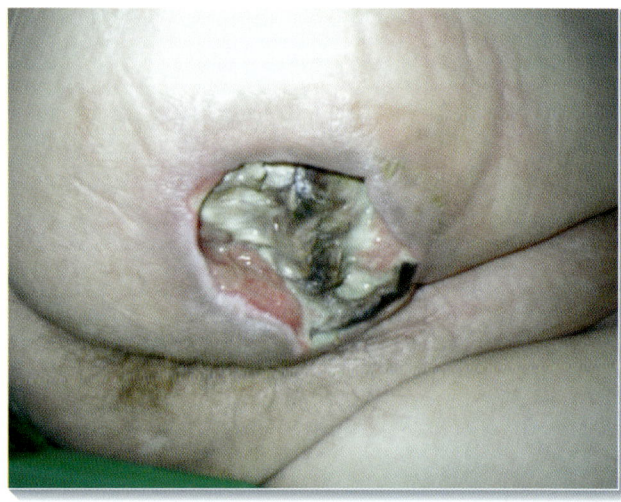

Figure 26.5 A wet environment.

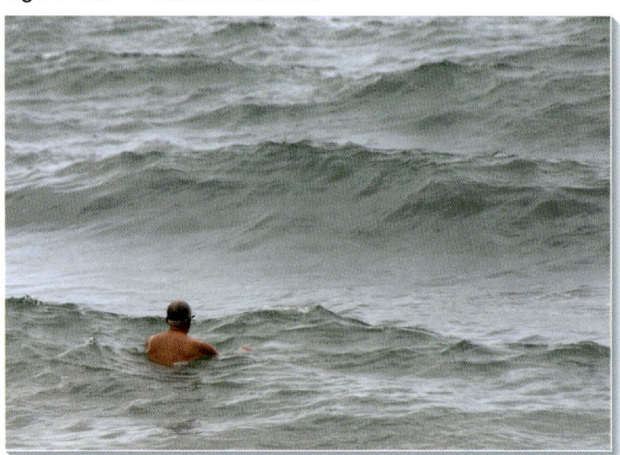

Source: iStock © cenix.

Figure 26.6 A wet wound environment.

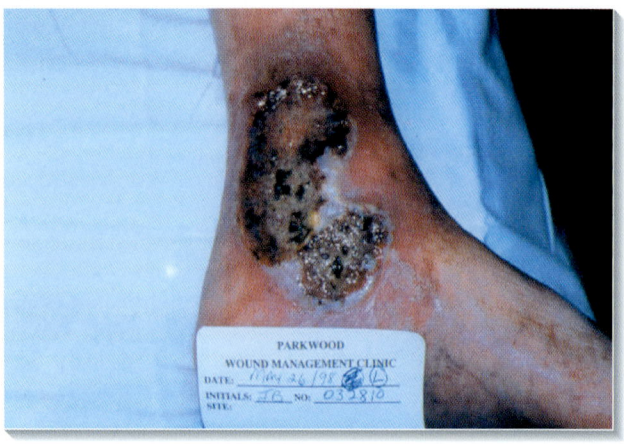

Source: Keast et al 2008, figure 9, S15. Reproduced with permission on Wiley & Sons Ltd.

Wound Care at a Glance, Second Edition. Ian Peate and Melanie Stephens.
© 2020 John Wiley & Sons Ltd. Published 2020 by John Wiley & Sons Ltd.
Companion website: http://www.ataglanceseries.com/nursing/woundcare/

Moist wound healing

A wound heals 50% faster in a moist environment as compared to the healing rates in a dry environment. Creating a moist wound environment facilitates all four phases of wound healing while minimising the growth of bacteria on the wound bed, thereby reducing the risk of wound infection.

During the healing phase, a moist wound decreases the intensity and duration of the inflammatory response, while trapping enzymes produced within the wound bed throughout the healing process. These enzymes facilitate autolytic debridement, which prevents the formation of debris on a wound bed (e.g. slough, necrosis and eschar). This, therefore, allows for easier and quicker migration of granulation and epithelial cells across the wound bed that would otherwise be obstructed by these barriers if the wound was dry and covered with debris. A moist environment naturally cleanses and irrigates the wound bed. A moist wound preserves the growth factors that are produced within the wound fluid, which assist with faster healing times. A moist wound increases the collagen synthesis and angiogenesis, and wound contraction occurs much quicker, thereby making for a more favourable cosmetic result during the maturation phase of wound healing. Throughout this process, bacteria find it much more difficult to multiply in a moist wound environment, as they favour either wet or dry environment depending on whether they are aerobic or anaerobic bacteria. A moist wound is therefore not favourable to either type of bacteria, and less likely to become infected. A moist wound also aids dressing removal and reduces pain without destroying newly formed tissue.

It is not possible to measure the amount of exudate present on a wound, or to specify the optimum amount to achieve the preceding benefits. However, it is possible to say that, in most cases, a 'moist' wound is preferred as opposed to a 'wet' or a 'dry' wound. So, how do we describe a moist wound? The following analogy may assist practitioners to recognise when a wound is moist, wet or dry, which can occur even when debris is present on the wound bed (i.e. necrosis, slough or eschar).

If you fall into a swimming pool, it does not matter how large or small that swimming pool is – you get completely wet. On the other hand, if you sit in the sand in the Sahara Desert, you get totally dry due to the absence of any moisture. Whereas, if you sit on an ice rink, you neither get wet nor dry; instead, you get 'damp' or 'moist'. It is the 'ice rink', damp environment that is equivalent to the optimum 'moist' wound environment that is aimed to be achieved in wound management (Figures 26.1, 26.2, 26.3, 26.4 and 26.5). This enables nurses to focus on the concept of wound bed preparation in order to encourage the normal processes of healing.

Let us now convert this analogy to the wet, dry or moist wound.

The wet wound

This type of wound requires frequent dressing changes due to saturation from excessive amounts of wound exudate (the volume of which is irrelevant, as it is either wet or it is not) (Figure 26.6). Often, there is visible exudate strike-through (staining) on the outer dressing, as the dressing reaches its maximum absorbing ability. The moisture is then be absorbed by the peri-wound skin, causing maceration (over hydration), which is white or silver in colour and may be wrinkly in appearance. If bacterial levels are high, as they are often in wet environments, the pH levels alter the exudate to a more acidic level that causes excoriation (burning) to the peri-wound skin, which is red in appearance. On dressing removal, exudate often runs off the wound.

The wet wound destroys the epithelial and granulation cells, and dilutes the growth factors, thereby stopping the wound from healing altogether in most cases. Infected wounds usually become wet, and exudate levels increase with increase in bacterial levels.

The dry wound

This wound is mostly dry and crusty, and has no sheen to it. There may be small patches of moisture present; however, it is considered a dry wound if the majority produces little or no exudate (Figure 26.4). The dressing should be dry and can often adhere to the wound (especially if a wrong dressing is selected). The patient often complains of a 'tightness' or pain on or around the wound. Any erythema (redness) around the wound is usually attributed to another cause, such as infection, the inflammatory response or the effects of pressure rather than from excoriation, and therefore requires further assessment.

It is difficult for granulation and epithelial cells to migrate across the dry wound bed, as the cells have to burrow under the dry debris. As a result of the obstruction, migrating cells are easily damaged and in doing so delay the healing process.

The moist wound

This wound appears 'damp' and glistens with moisture, although no moisture appears to drip from the wound (Figure 26.2). There is no evidence of maceration or excoriation (unless from some other cause, as previously stated), as exudate levels are managed adequately in the dressing, which is changed immediately if any exudate strike-through appears. On average, this dressing requires changing once, twice or three times per week, depending on the size and depth of the wound and stage of wound healing.

It is unusual for a moist wound to become infected, provided these moisture levels are maintained. In the case of an infection, it no longer remains a moist wound and becomes a wet one instead.

Managing wound exudate

The optimum moist environment pushes for faster healing rates, as previously described. In order to achieve this, it is vital that the most appropriate dressing is selected in the first instance, and timely dressing changes are carried out in the second. Dressing changes must be dictated by the levels of exudate (i.e. by evidence of strike-through) rather than an estimate of time (e.g. change every 3 days).

27 Generic wound products: mode of action

Table 27.1 A summary of different types of dressings.

Generic dressing type	Common brands in each category	Indications	Contraindications	Cautions	Type of wound
Hydrocolloid	Granuflex Duoderm, Hydrocoll Comfeel, Tegaderm hydrcolloid, Ultec Pro, ActivHeal, Askina Biofilm, Flexigran, Nu-Derm	Dry or low exuding wounds	Heavily exuding (wet) wounds, Infected wounds, Any risk of gas gangrene	Diabetic foot ulcers	Pressure ulcers, Leg ulcers, Surgical wounds, Dehisced wounds, Traumatic wounds, Ruptured blisters
Foams – Polyurethane, Hydrocellular, Soft silicone, Hydropolymer (adhesive or non-adhesive)	Biatain, Lyofoam, Allevyn, Mepilex, ActivHeal, Kendall Island, PermaFoam, Tegaderm Foam, Tielle, PolyMem	Moist, moderate or heavily exuding wounds (i.e. moist to wet)	None	Sensitivities: Avoid direct applications to dry wounds (unless that is the aim – discussed in other chapters) Avoid direct contact with intact skin as far as possible to prevent dehydration	All wound types
Deodorising	CarboFlex, Actisorb Silver 200, CliniSorb, LyofoamC, Carbonet	Malodorous wounds	Dry wounds	Avoid direct applications to dry wounds. Some are ineffective when wet	Fungating and malodorous wounds
Film	Hydrofilm, C-View, Tegaderm, Opsite, Mepitel Film, Mepore Film, Askina Derm, Dressfilm, Hypafix, Lukomed T, Polyskin II, Protectfilm, Suprasorb F	On fragile, vulnerable skin with no exudate, or on low exuding wounds if an alginate or hydrofibre is applied to the wound first	None	None	Superficial wounds of all types and on vulnerable skin or scar tissue
Alginates	Sorbsan–Kaltostat, ActivHeal, Algisite M, Algosteril, Biatain Alginate, Cutimed Alginate, Kendall, Melgisorb, Sorbalgon, Suprasorb A, Tegaderm Alginate	For all wounds with any level of moisture. Can be moistened by 20% if the wound is dry	None	Sensitivities: Must be covered with an insulating dressing	All wound types. Not suitable if the wound is to be completely dried out, as it will remain moist
Hydrocolloid fibrous	Aquacel (plain), Aquacel Foam, UrgoClean pad/rope	For all wounds with any level of moisture. Can be moistened by 20%, if the wound is dry	None	Sensitivities: Must be covered with an insulating dressing	All wound types. Not suitable if the wound is to be completely dried out, as it will remain moist

Wound Care at a Glance, Second Edition. Ian Peate and Melanie Stephens.
© 2020 John Wiley & Sons Ltd. Published 2020 by John Wiley & Sons Ltd.
Companion website: http://www.ataglanceseries.com/nursing/woundcare/

Generic dressing type	Common brands in each category	Indications	Contraindications	Cautions	Type of wound
Hydrogel	Actiheal, Aquaform, Askina, Cutimed, Flexigran, Granugel, Intrasite, Nu-gel, Purilon	For dry or very low exuding wounds	Heavily exuding (wet) wounds, Infected wounds, Any risk of gas gangrene	Diabetic foot ulcers	All wound types
Hydrogel sheet	ActiFormCool (sheet), Aquaflo, Coolie, Gel FX, Geliperm, Hydrosorb, Intrasite, Novogel, SanoSkin, VacuNet				
Low-adherent	Silicone or knitted fabrics, Atrauman, N-A, Mepitel, Profore, Tricotex, UrgoTul, Cuticell, Jelonet, Neotulle, ParaGauze, Paranet	To prevent dressings adhering to a wound	None	May not achieve the aim of a moist wound-healing environment	All wound types
Other dressing types	Absorbent pad, for example, Kerramax, Eclypse Surgipads, Gamgee, gauze, dressing pads	With the exception of highly absorbent pads, there is very minimal place for this type of dressing in modern wound care	Not advisable for open wounds unless for exudate management of non-healing wounds	Does not insulate a wound and has a tendency to dry a wound out, causing adherence. Some Gamgees are treated with bleach	Not recommended on any wound type, except wet, non-healing wounds, such as leg ulcers, until such time the causes of exudate levels are addressed and levels reduce

Wound products

It is essential that any product chosen for use on a wound be selected on the basis of the clinical assessment of the wound and the holistic assessment of the patient and in accordance with the aims that the nurse is trying to achieve.

It is essential that the products used on a wound be prescribed; however, because most nurses are not authorised to prescribe, it is common for dressings to be selected from a 'dressings formulary'. This is a list of wound care dressing products that have been scrutinised and approved by an organisation for use on wounds, and therefore negates the need for each and every product on that formulary to be prescribed. The nurse is therefore supported legally if she/he selects a product from a formulary, provided she/he uses it for the purposes it is intended.

Let us now consider typical generic products that are found on a dressing's formulary; their mode of action; when to use them and when they are contraindicated on wounds (Table 27.1).

- *Hydrocolloids*: These are hydrating products that can be used on dry wounds with little or no moisture in order to raise the exudate levels to a moist environment. They must be changed immediately if there is an evidence of strike-through in order to avoid saturation and therefore, maceration or excoriation that could quickly lead to infection. Once the wound reaches the optimum 'moist' level, consideration must be given to the wear time of this dressing and whether or not it remains appropriate, as it then requires more frequent dressing changes if its use continues. This product is an 'insulating' product, meaning that it maintains body temperature on the wound bed and can be used alone as the primary dressing or as a secondary dressing with alginates or hydrofibres underneath. Contraindications are listed in Table 27.1 and discussed in other chapters.
- *Foams*: These are absorbent dressings intended to reduce exudate levels. However, these products, if used alone, could potentially dry the wound out completely, as they absorb exudate faster than the body can produce it. In order to avoid drying, alginates or hydrofibrous dressings can be used underneath to maintain a moist environment. They are insulating dressings, thereby maintaining body temperature on the wound. Contraindications are listed in Table 27.1 and discussed in other chapters.
- *Deodorising*: These products contain a charcoal cloth that is able to absorb gas molecules. Some deodorising dressings are

combined with other dressing products, such as foam, silver, alginates and absorbent pads. It is important to check if the charcoal becomes ineffective when wet from exudate.

- *Films*: These products neither absorb moisture nor hydrate wounds. Used on their own, they can only be used on vulnerable but unbroken skin (e.g. a Grade 1 pressure damage, areas vulnerable to friction or on healed wounds that require some protection for a while). Films can be used with either an alginate or a hydrofibre placed underneath and together this combination can be used on low to moderate exuding wounds. Films insulate the wound, thereby maintaining body temperature.
- *Alginates*: These are absorbent primary dressings that require one of the aforementioned insulating secondary dressings applied over them. The failure in 'insulating' this type of dressing causes it to dry and adhere to the wound bed, thereby causing trauma on removal. This type of dressing is required for deeper wounds in order to 'fill' them to skin level. They can also be applied to shallower wounds in order to assist with maintaining a 'moist' wound and to increase the absorbency and therefore the wear time of the dressing.
- *Hydrofibrous*: This is an absorbent primary dressing that also maintains a moist wound environment if an insulating primary dressing is applied over it. It is used in the same way that an alginate is used; however, it is considered by some as having the additional benefit of trapping bacteria, as it absorbs wound exudate.
- *Hydrogels/hydrogel sheets*: These are hydrating products intended to raise the moisture levels of a dry wound to 'moist'. Hydrogels consist of approximately 20% polysaccharides and 80% water, thereby producing a watery gel, whereas, hydrogel sheets consist of approximately 20% water and 80% polysaccharides, enabling a thicker consistency and thereby forming a sheet. A gel sheet absorbs some moisture within the polysaccharides, but the liquid gel does not absorb anything. Care must be taken when selecting a secondary dressing, because to apply a liquid gel to a wound covered by a foam, for example, negates the effects intended by the gel, as it is absorbed into the dressing.
- *Non-adherent*: These are dressings that do not insulate the wound, neither hydrate nor absorb moisture and are commonly used for superficial wounds under other dressing types to prevent them from adhering to the wound. Many wound experts consider that these dressing types have little usefulness in wound care and are therefore most frequently used with vacuum-assisted closure treatments (topical negative pressure) and will be discussed later.
- *Other dressing types*: This category includes dressing types specifically designed to provide combinations of the dressing types discussed in the preceding text – for example, a combination of a hydrofibre and a hydrocolloid. Alternatively, such dressings as highly absorbent pads, Gamgee, dressing pads and other common products are selected for their cost-effectiveness, or when the aim of the wound is to manage wound exudate when there is no prospect of wound healing based on underlying factors. Many experts consider that the use of these products is limited due to their lack of wound insulation.
- *Antimicrobials*: Currently, there are three main categories of antimicrobial dressings; silver, honey and iodine impregnated dressings. Honey and iodine also come in a paste or an ointment that is often applied to wounds under appropriate dressings. Selection of a particular antimicrobial depends on the products available to the nurse on the dressing's formulary and based on a holistic wound assessment. Antimicrobials will be discussed in greater detail in later chapters.

Dressing selection depends on many things and it is important that nurses have a sound knowledge of each dressing type available and the dressing's mode of action. It is important that the nurse responsible for wound care be fully aware of the indications and contraindications for use in order to appropriately apply a dressing's formulary. Inappropriate selection of the dressing can cause harm to the patient.

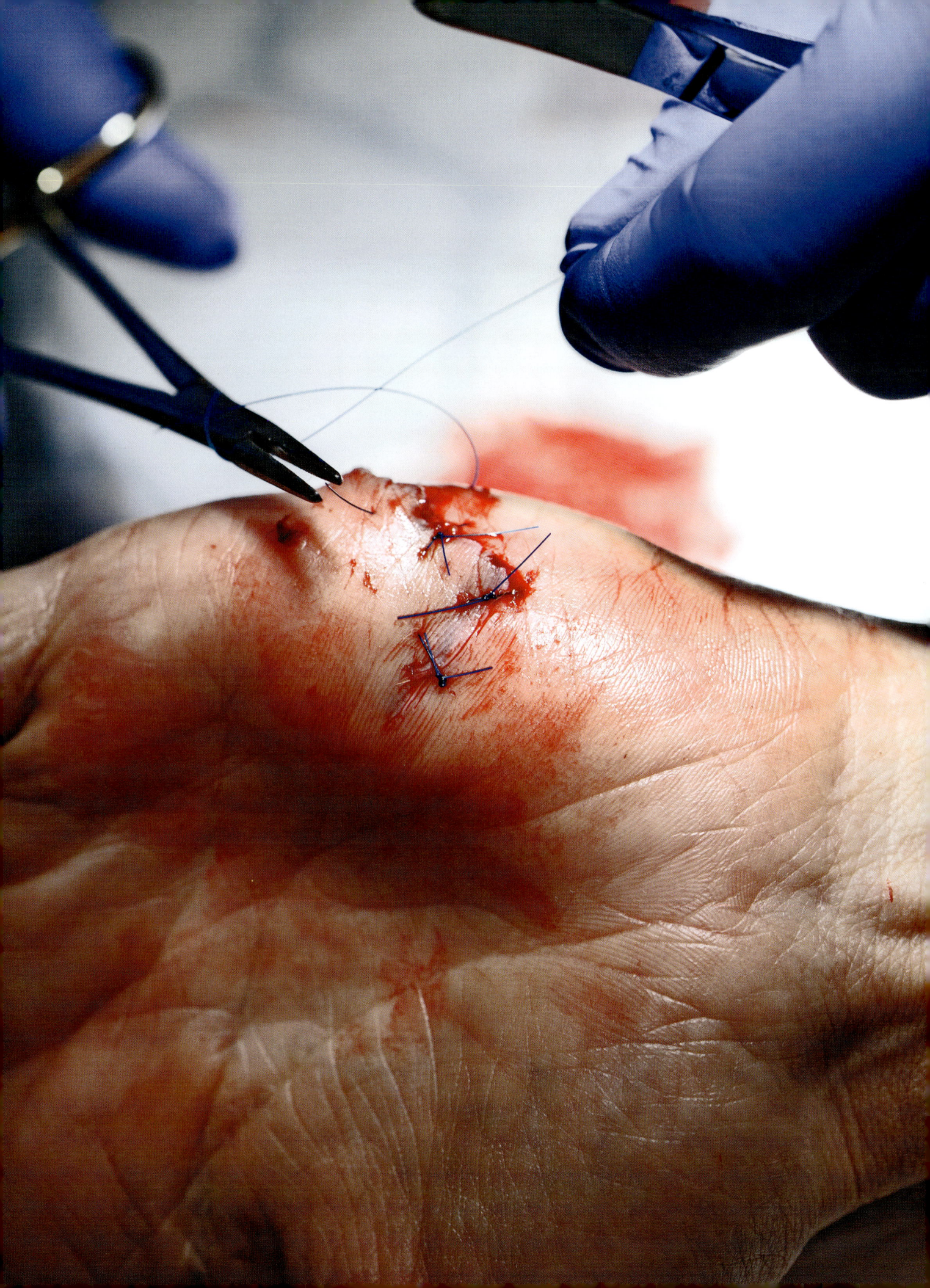

28 Choosing a wound care product

Figure 28.1 (i–iv) Dressing Selection Guide.

Clinical observation	What is happening at the cellular level?	Wound bed preparation (WBP)	Expected outcome of WBP	Clinical goal
Tissue is non-viable 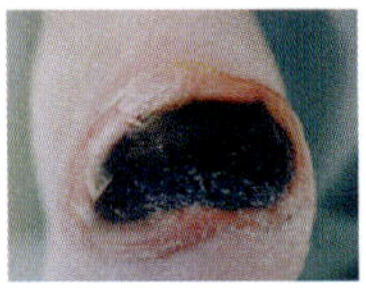	Malfunctioning matrix and cell debris impairing wound healing	Debridement of the wound via autolytic, sharp, surgical, enzymatic or biological agents	Restoration of wound bed and functional extracellular matrix	Viable wound bed
Infection or Inflammation 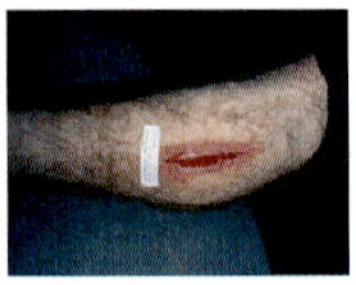	Critical colonisation, biofilm or infection	Remove infected foci with topical antimicrobials, systemic/topical antibiotics* and anti-inflammatories	Lower the bacterial count, which decreases exudate production, odour, pain, swelling, redness and heat	Bacterial balance
Moisture 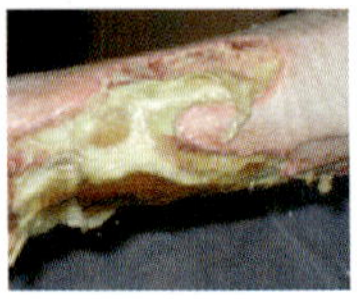	Dry wound bed delays epithelial cell migration, and excess exudate causes maceration	Restore moisture balance through either hydration (adding moisture to wound) or managing wound exudate (compression, NWPT and absorbent dressings)	Restore moist wound environment and reduce risk of infection, maceration and delayed wound healing	Moisture balance
Edge of the wound 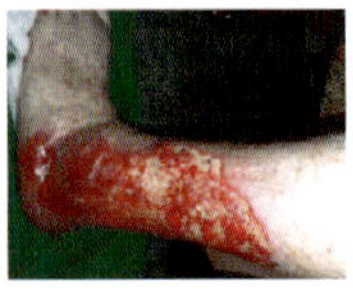	Assess for the non-migration of epithelial cells, delayed contraction of the wound edges, signs of maceration/excoriation/dryness and damage from dressing removal or allergy	Assess the cause and apply appropriate dressing, such as moisture balance, barrier film/cream and patch test for allergy; reassess the primary dressing choice	Restore wound bed, so that the cells migrate for wound contraction, manage exudate, hydrate dry skin and provide protection	Advancing wound edge

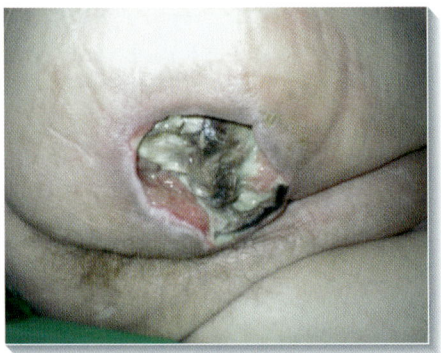

Figure 28.2   Week 1.

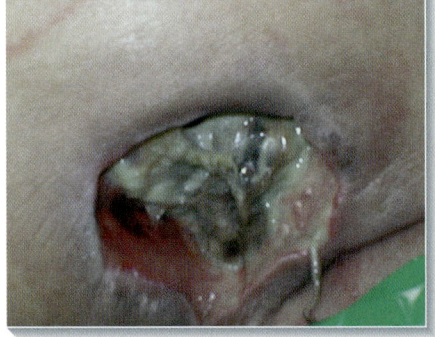

Figure 28.3   Week 3.

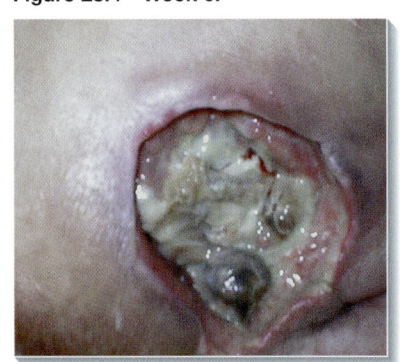

Figure 28.4   Week 6.

Wound Care at a Glance, Second Edition. Ian Peate and Melanie Stephens.
© 2020 John Wiley & Sons Ltd. Published 2020 by John Wiley & Sons Ltd.
Companion website: http://www.ataglanceseries.com/nursing/woundcare/

Aims in wound care

The aim in wound management is to achieve a 'moist' wound-healing environment in most cases (exceptions to moist healing will be discussed in later chapters). Moist wound healing can be achieved by the application of modern wound dressings, accompanied by timely dressing changes to prevent saturation. If this moisture level is achieved, it assists with the preparation of the wound bed so that the wound heals as promptly as it possibly can.

As part of this process, it is important to assess the wound in detail in order to (a) ensure that the most appropriate product/treatment is selected, and (b) to devise an appropriate plan of care for the ongoing management and monitoring of the wound. Although there are many aspects to consider when assessing a wound, many nurses utilise a framework known as TIME in order to systematically consider relevant issues before applying a treatment. This is explained in the following text.

Tissue, Infection, Moisture, Edge (TIME)

- *Tissue*: The nurse makes note of the types of tissues on the wound bed. The tissues that may require removal can be the dead and devitalised tissues (such as necrosis) or unwanted debris (such as slough, dead skin or foreign bodies), all of which can inhibit healing rates while creating a harbour for bacterial growth. Consideration must be given to the most appropriate method to remove unwanted tissues. This could be achieved by autolytic debridement, by the use of larval therapy (maggots), by sharp debridement by a nurse trained in the technique or by surgical debridement under anaesthetic by a surgeon.
- *Infection*: The nurse observes the wound and the surrounding skin and tissues for any signs of infection. High levels of bacteria usually produce high levels of exudate, and this could be the only indication that bacterial levels on a wound are high. A wet wound in the absence of two or more clinical signs of infection is regarded as heavily (or critically) colonised wound and not infected. Treatment choice depends on whether or not an infection is clinically identified.
- *Moisture*: Moisture levels on a wound can vary from light to heavy within hours, for a variety of reasons (e.g. bacteria levels, leaking oedema, hydrating products, etc.). The nurse must therefore continually assess the moisture levels oozing from a wound in order to select the most appropriate dressing product to manage it. Failure to do so allows excess moisture onto the wound and surrounding tissues, which causes maceration, thereby hindering healing while creating an optimum environment for rapid bacterial growth and increasing the risk of infection.
- *Edge*: The nurse must observe the edges of the wound for signs of healing (by granulation, epithelialisation and wound shrinkage by maturation), as well as for signs of infection and/or damage to surrounding tissues caused by maceration or excoriation from poorly contained moisture levels, or from damage or allergy to products used. Any untoward signs can determine what product should or should not to be used on the wound.

Dressing selection guide

Once the nurse assesses the wound and surrounding skin/tissues, it is essential that she/he records this on a wound assessment chart. These findings in conjunction with the findings on holistic assessment of the patient enable the nurse to identify the aims of care required to remove unwanted tissue (if any); avoid the production of unwanted tissue; promote healing while eradicating/preventing infection and/or damage to healthy tissues by appropriately managing exudate levels, all of which must be included in a care plan that can direct others on the management of the wound to achieve these aims.

The dressing selection guide shown in Figure 28.1(i–iv) can assist the nurse in selecting the most appropriate product once the patient and his/her wound is fully assessed, by considering the clinical findings to reach the most appropriate treatment option.

Case study

Mr. Joe Bloggs is an 83-year-old multiple sclerosis patient who sustained a Category 4 pressure ulcer while undergoing a prostatectomy. He has no other medical history; he is mentally competent, communicates verbally, has no allergies and is fully dependent on others for all activities of daily living. He has a normal range body mass index and is otherwise reasonably healthy with good immunity. His wound is sited over the right ischial tuberosity (sitting bones). Using TIME, an assessment of the wound shown in Figure 28.2 divulges the following clinical findings:

- *T*: The tissues on the wound bed consist of approximately 85% slough and 15% healthy granulation tissues.
- *I*: There is no evidence of infection (no surrounding erythema, pus, dry to minimal exudate, no malodour or pain and no friable wound bed).
- *M*: Moisture levels are minimal (confirmed by the absence of maceration or excoriation to the surrounding skin), and the dressing was not saturated on removal after 6 days.
- *E*: Edges of the wound are healthy: no maceration, excoriation, trauma or allergic reactions.

Using the dressing selection guide

Based on the holistic wound findings, effective pressure redistribution was provided, and it was agreed that the patient's health and immunity were sufficient to withstand active autolytic debridement (discussed later) by way of hydrofibrous dressing rather than by passive autolytic debridement (also discussed later) or surgical intervention. Hydrofibrous dressings were stopped once the wound had become moist (Figure 28.3), and passive autolytic debridement was adopted thereafter until the wound was fully healed. Figure 28.4 shows the wound almost fully debrided, but with a significantly shallower wound depth, which came about by allowing granulation tissue to fill the wound in the moist environment that was maintained throughout. The surrounding skin was healthy throughout, and there were no wound infection events during the process.

29 Use of topical antimicrobials and antibiotics

Figure 29.1 The level of bacterial growth on a wound and the effect on healing.

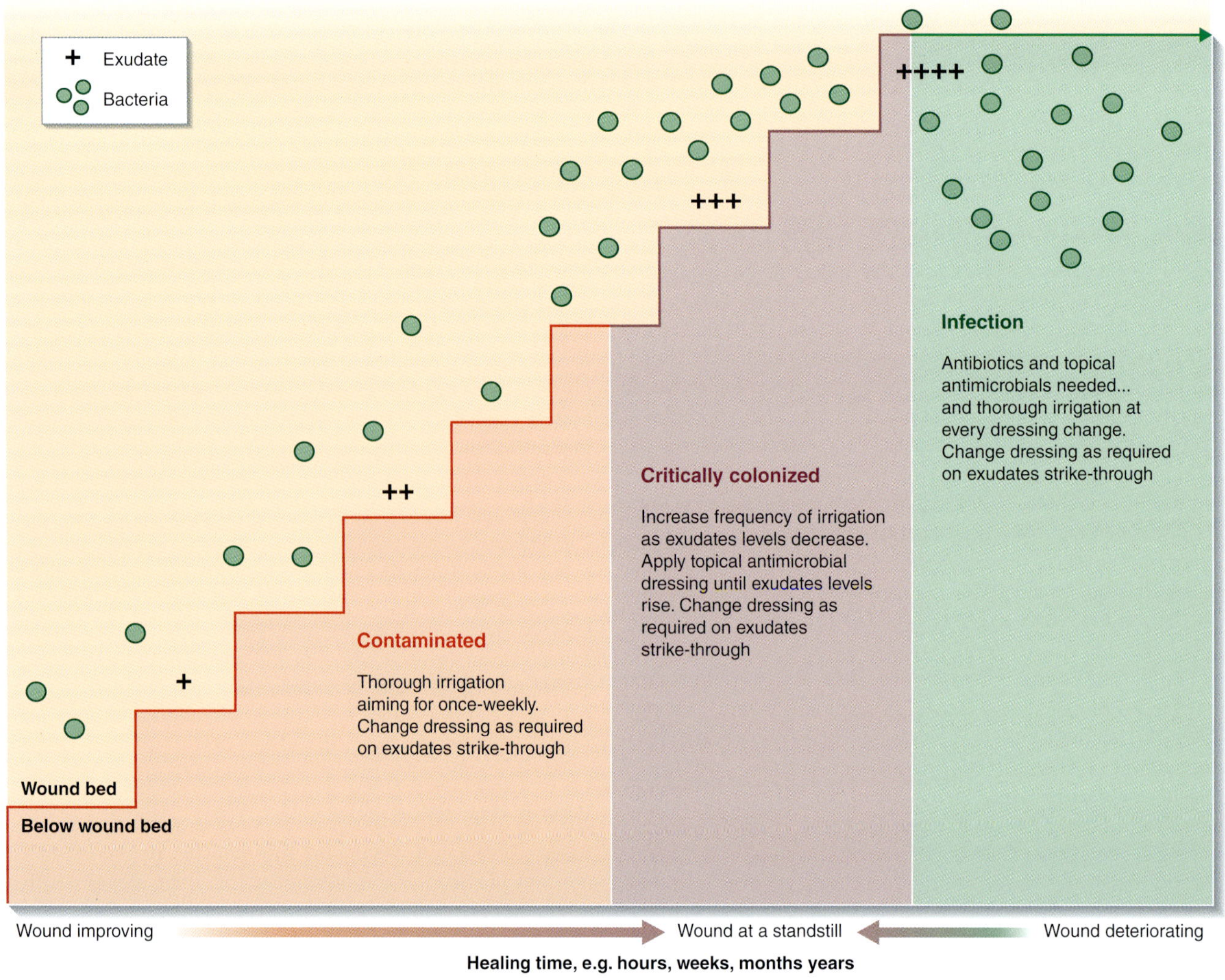

- **+** Exudate
- **○** Bacteria

Contaminated
Thorough irrigation aiming for once-weekly. Change dressing as required on exudates strike-through

Critically colonized
Increase frequency of irrigation as exudates levels decrease. Apply topical antimicrobial dressing until exudates levels rise. Change dressing as required on exudates strike-through

Infection
Antibiotics and topical antimicrobials needed... and thorough irrigation at every dressing change. Change dressing as required on exudates strike-through

Wound bed / Below wound bed

Wound improving → Wound at a standstill ← Wound deteriorating

Healing time, e.g. hours, weeks, months years

Wound Care at a Glance, Second Edition. Ian Peate and Melanie Stephens.
© 2020 John Wiley & Sons Ltd. Published 2020 by John Wiley & Sons Ltd.
Companion website: http://www.ataglanceseries.com/nursing/woundcare/

The skin is contaminated with bacteria, which are usually harmless; however, when a wound occurs there is a possibility that microbes can cause an infection, as the natural protective mechanism of the skin gets broken down. The presence of microbes in the wound is categorised into levels: contaminated, colonised, critically colonised and infected (see Figure 29.1). Contaminated wounds do not tend to increase bacteria load or cause clinical effect; colonised wounds contain multiplying microbes but again these do not damage or effect wound-healing processes. Critical colonisation happens when the wound moves from containing multiplying bacteria to an infected state with impaired healing; however, there is no invasion of the tissues and no signs of an inflammatory response. Infection occurs when the bacteria multiply, invade and damaging tissues, causing a local or systemic response (sepsis). Prior to making a final decision on the level of contamination in the wound bed, a nurse must also consider the possibility of a biofilm. A biofilm is a complex community of one or several types of bacteria that develop on or near a wound surface. They are invisible to the naked eye, but on assessment of the wound, the patient may present with a chronic non-healing or impaired wound healing.

Once a diagnosis of a spreading infection or biofilm at the wound site is made, the appropriate treatment is necessary. Prior to deciding on the type of treatment and dressing products required, a full assessment of both the patient and the wound is essential. Using the TIME framework assists in examining the viability of the tissue at the wound bed, the signs and symptoms of infection, moisture imbalance and edges of the wound.

From best practice statements, clinicians should initially clean the wound using a non-touch technique and then choose the most appropriate treatment and dressing. This should vary depending on whether the diagnosis is wound infection or biofilm. With an infected wound, a patient requires systemic antibiotics, and, depending on the local policy, a topical antimicrobial dressing may be required. These dressings ought to be applied to the wound bed to assist in reducing bacterial levels on the wound, which reduces the risk of reinfection once systemic antibiotics eliminate the infection under the wound bed.

Topical antimicrobials, while reducing the bacterial bioburden on the wound bed, do not eliminate a spreading infection. The risk of infection can be reduced if bacterial levels on the wound are kept to a minimum, as it is most commonly the high number of bacteria (of any species) living on the wound bed rather than specific species that is important in the treatment of most infections. Control of bacterial growth can be better achieved by maintaining a 'moist' wound-healing environment; by thorough irrigation of the wound bed at appropriate intervals and by the use of topical antimicrobial dressings and other wound treatment products when they are required. Figure 29.1 gives guidance on when to use each of these methods of control.

Biofilms, however, require an alternative action after wound irrigation. Best practices suggest that biofilms require debridement or robust physical cleansing, and even the use of topical antiseptic agents. However, it is always best to check your local policy, and ensure you have the appropriate training, knowledge and skills to carry out this procedure. The nurse should never attempt biofilm debridement on patients with severe vascular compromise. It should be remembered that there are always other members of the interprofessional team and dressing products in the wound care tool box that can help in debriding a wound safely (wound care specialists, surgeons, podiatrists, larvae, dressings, etc.).

Common antimicrobials

There are different types of antimicrobial products available. The following text will discuss the pros and cons of each product. The selection of a particular product depends on the findings of a holistic wound assessment, the level of contamination (signs and symptoms of critical colonisation/infection), the patient's ability to fight bacterial invasion and the products that are accessible to the health professionals, who usually selects a product from a wound dressing formulary agreed within their organisation. There are only two situations where antimicrobials should be used: when signs and symptoms suggest that wound bioburden is impeding on wound healing, and in case of an increased risk of serious outcomes. Once started, the effect of the antimicrobial dressing should be monitored closely, and a full review conducted every 2 weeks. The review should include an assessment of the progression of wound healing and infection; these findings assist in determining whether the antimicrobial should stop, continue for a further two weeks or change to a different approach. All findings should be documented clearly, and timely referral to other members of the interprofessional team should be made.

Enzyme alginogel

An alginate gel that contains two antibacterial enzymes is used in acute and chronic wounds to promote autolytic debridement, maintain moisture balance, decrease the number of bacteria in the wound bed and protect wound edges and epithelial cells. The product is also safe to use on pregnant women, as there is no absorption into the body. The alginate gel is usually applied to the wound bed and covered with a secondary dressing. It requires regular dressing checks to ensure the correct level of gel and can be used long term. Contraindications include using dressings with known allergies to alginates dressing or polyethylene glycol. Alginate gels should not to be used near the eyes.

Honey and honey-impregnated dressings

Medical-grade honey has antimicrobial and anti-inflammatory properties, and can be used for acute or chronic wounds. Honey has osmotic properties that produce an environment that promotes autolytic debridement (i.e. the removal of debris on the wound bed). As it kills and reduces bacterial levels, malodour and pain are reduced in turn. It is a reasonably cost-effective product and is effective on a large number of bacterial species. The mode of delivery is via gel, ointment, impregnated dressing, gel sheet or cream.

The disadvantage of using honey is that not all bacteria are eradicated with its use, and, in fact, some bacteria are known to thrive on the sugar found in honey. As honey has an osmotic effect, the end product is H_2O (water), which can make a wound wet. This situation can be conducive for rapid bacterial growth, and, as there is no sustained release of antimicrobial product, the wet environment could lead to reinfection. It is therefore vital that the dressing is closely observed for exudate strike-through (staining on the outer/secondary dressing), and that it is changed before it becomes saturated. The increased dressing changes and risk of reinfection could negate any savings made on using this cheaper antimicrobial. Finally, care must be taken when using this product on patients who are diabetic, and regular blood sugar checks must be made. Care must also be taken when using this product on those with known hypersensitivities to bee stings. The product should not be used on full-thickness burns.

Iodine and iodine-impregnated dressings

This product is commonly chosen as a first-line antimicrobial, because it is cheap to purchase. The two main types of iodine are:

1 *Cadexomer iodine* is placed in ointments and pastes. This enables the release of free iodine when exposed to wound exudate. This serves as an antiseptic on the wound surface. It can absorb exudate and aid desloughing of wound debris. Common products in this category are Iodoflex and Iodosorb. The disadvantage of iodine is that it has a known (and increasing) bacterial resistance; systemic absorption of iodine can occur if applied to a large wound or used for prolonged periods, and should therefore only be used in accordance with directions in the British National Formulary (BNF). It is contraindicated for children, pregnant and breast-feeding women, for those with thyroid conditions and those who are prescribed lithium. As it is absorbed, it is difficult to achieve a sustained release of antimicrobial, which means that reinfection can easily occur.

2 *Povidone iodine* is impregnated into a knitted viscose dressing incorporated in a hydrophilic polyethylene glycol base that facilitates diffusion of the iodine onto the wound bed. It has a wide spectrum of antimicrobial activity; however, this is rapidly deactivated on contact with wound exudate. An example that is commonly used is Inadine. Disadvantages of this product are mentioned in the preceding text, and it is difficult to achieve a sustained release of antimicrobials, as the iodine is deactivated with wound exudate; therefore, reinfection can easily occur.

Silver-impregnated dressings

Silver has a broad spectrum of antimicrobial activity and has, to date, no known bacterial resistance. The volume of wound exudate must be considered when choosing a silver dressing. There are two types of silver products available.

1 *Silver metallic, nanocrystalline or ionic products* that are present within dressings and pastes are used to manage wound bioburden and provide an antimicrobial. They are used on both acute and chronic wounds, and in some paediatric wounds. The dressings are generally applied direct to the wound, some have to be moistened to activate the release of silver. Most are used for 2 weeks, and, after review, these can be used for a further 2 weeks or discontinued. Long-term use can increase the risk of argyria (the build-up of silver in the body, turning the tissues purple or purplish grey). Contraindications include use on wounds of large surface area, patients with sensitivity to silver, pregnant and breast-feeding women and avoid using when a patient is undergoing an MRI scan or radiotherapy.

2 *Silver sulphadiazine*: This is a cream or an impregnated dressing containing silver salts used for the prevention of infection in burns, leg ulcers and pressure ulcers. The product is initially used for 1 week. The cream should be applied with 0.3–0.5 cm thickness. In case of no improvement, it can be used for up to 2 weeks. Long-term use can increase the risk of argyria. Contraindications include avoiding its use on patients with sensitivity to silver and children under 2 months of age. Care should be taken with pregnant and breast-feeding women and patients with liver and renal disease.

This product may be absorbed, causing blood disorders and skin discolouration. Other silver dressings can be of the metallic or ionic silver types, neither of which is absorbed, so there are no contraindications for their use. People with an allergy to metallic silver may be at risk of a reaction; however, provided the dressing containing metallic silver is not in contact with the skin and only with wound exudate, the metal aspect gets converted to ionic silver in a chemical reaction with the exudate. Till date, there is no known allergy to ionic silver, and it is not absorbed. The disadvantage of silver products is their cost. However, if they are chosen carefully, they can be left in situ on the wound for a number of days, thereby changing only the outer dressing and reducing costs.

Octenidine solution, cream and gel

Octenidine is prepared as a solution, cream and gel that contain the active substances, octenidine dihydrochloride and phenoxyethanol, which have antiseptic properties. It is used for two weeks to either clean and decontaminate the skin or a wound, manage a bioburden, remove necrotic tissues or hydrate the tissue or skin. It is used in both acute and chronic wounds, including paediatric wounds. This product is applied directly to the skin or wound bed, and the nurse should wait for 2 minutes before applying a secondary dressing. The solution is left on for 5 minutes, and can be used to soften dressings before removal. Contraindications include those patients who are allergic to octenidine dihydrochloride and phenoxyethanol. Not to be used on patients with exposed joint or cartilage, in abdominal cavities, ears (outer, inner and drum) and eyes.

Polyhexamethylene biguanide

Dressings, gels and solutions containing polyhexamethylene biguanide (PHMB) are used because of the presence of a synthetic antiseptic agent, which disrupts the cell membranes and metabolism of bacteria, interfering with function and causing cell death. These are used to cleanse and decontaminate wounds, assist in removing encrusted dressings (solution), curb biofilm formation, manage wound bioburden, reduce wound odour and provide an antimicrobial barrier. Their use is mainly for partial-thickness burns, postsurgical wounds, traumatic wounds, skin donor/recipient sites, leg ulcers, pressure ulcers, diabetic foot ulcers, scleroderma wounds and paediatric wounds. The solution (used at room temperature or warmed) should be applied for 15 minutes, and there is no need for rinsing off the solution afterwards. The gel can be applied directly to the wound bed, including areas of tunnelling and cavities. A secondary dressing is required and can be left in place for 5–7 days. Contraindications include known PHMB sensitivity, not to be combined with other wound cleansers or ointments, should be used with caution under medical supervision in pregnant and lactating women, and babies. PHMB is not to be used in peritoneal, joint, ears, central nervous system and eye lavage.

Dialkyl carbamoyl chloride

Dialkyl carbamoyl chloride (DACC)–coated dressings are produced in a variety of primary wound contact layers (ribbon, round swabs, absorbent pads, foams, hydropolymer gel matrix, etc.). The product is designed to permanently bind and inactivate bacteria and fungi, reducing the number of bacteria in moist wounds without releasing chemicals into the wound bed. The dressings absorb exudate and debride sloughy wounds. The product is prescribed to be used in treating patients with pressure ulcers, leg ulcers, diabetic foot wounds, traumatic and postoperatively dehisced surgical wounds, sinus and cavity wounds, burns and overgranulated wounds. The dressings can be used by children and pregnant women. They often require no further secondary dressing and can be secured with tape, retention bandage or stockinette. Dressing changes are as needed and should not be longer than 7 days. Contraindications of this product include not to be used in combination with other ointments and creams, as binding effect might be impaired.

Absorbent cellulose fibre gelling agents

These dressings are used to debride the slough autolytically, absorb exudate and remove bacteria and fungi from the wound bed. They are designed for use in moderate to heavily exuding wounds by applying the dressing directly to the wound bed, and require changing according to exudate levels and strike-through. The only contraindication is to avoid use on wounds with little or no exudate.

Topical antibiotics must be avoided unless directed by a specialist, as the antibiotic is usually impregnated into a gel or a cream. As the infected wound is usually a 'wet' wound, the antibiotic is diluted and absorbed into the dressing, so that there is no sustained release of the antibiotic. This leads to bacterial resistance to that antibiotic.

30 Application of lotions, creams, emollients and ointments

Figure 30.1 The Dermol range of emollients.

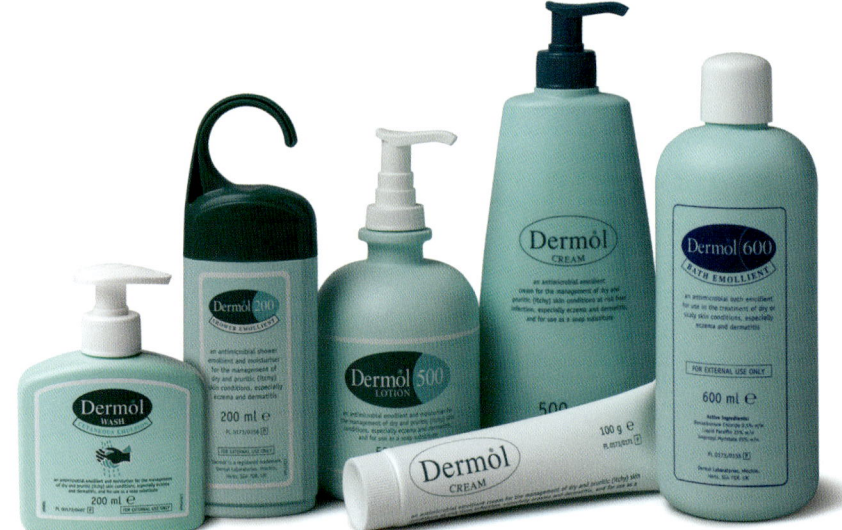

Source: Dermal Laboratories Ltd. Reproduced with permission of Dermal Laboratories Ltd.

Figure 30.2 Epaderm cream, which is used to manage skin conditions such as eczema and psoriasis.

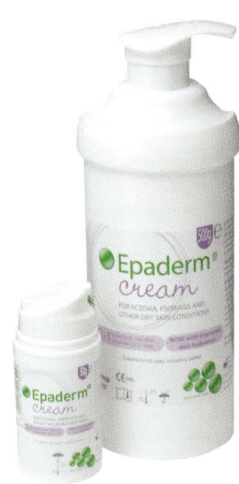

Source: Mölnlycke Health Care. Reproduced with permission of Mölnlycke Health Care.

Figure 30.3 The Cavilon range of barrier products, which act to protect the skin from excess moisture, for example, from body fluids.

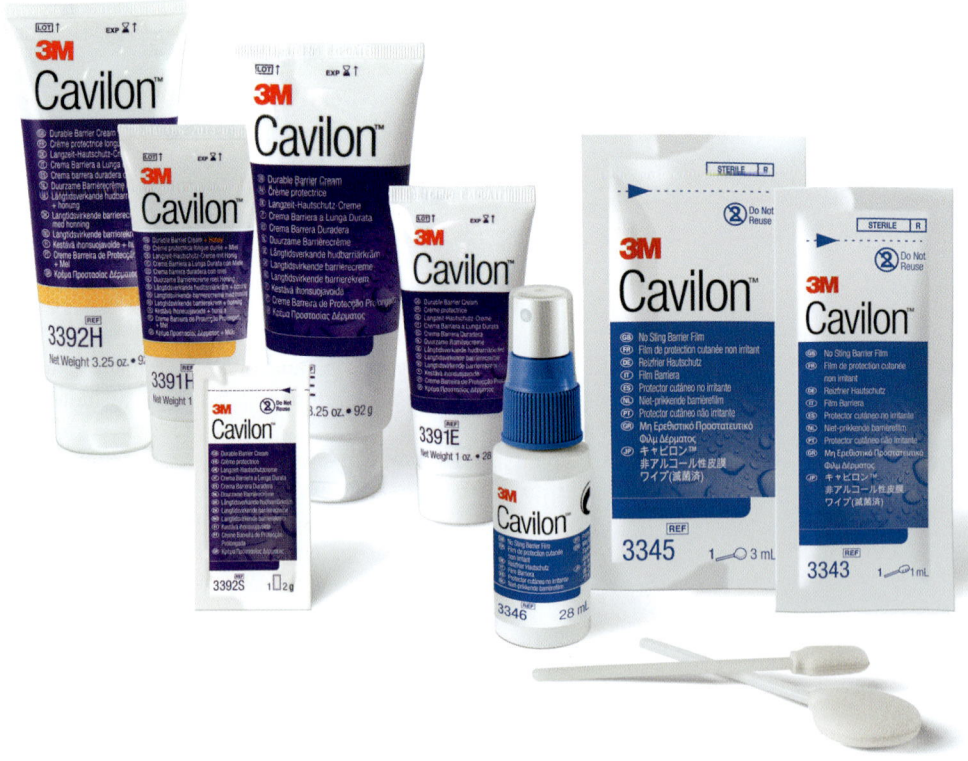

Source: Image © 3M. Reproduced with permission of 3M.

Wound Care at a Glance, Second Edition. Ian Peate and Melanie Stephens.
© 2020 John Wiley & Sons Ltd. Published 2020 by John Wiley & Sons Ltd.
Companion website: http://www.ataglanceseries.com/nursing/woundcare/

Appropriate and effective skin care is a vital part of maintaining tissue viability, particularly with ageing, because of slower cell regeneration. It is particularly important to care for the skin in order to protect it from moisture damage. Moisture damage can occur from sweating, particularly on skin folds, from incontinence of urine and faeces and around peri-wound skin from wound exudate.

The skin is affected by external conditions, such as low humidity and by excessive bathing using soaps and other products that can strip it of natural oils (sebum), causing it to dry. Smoking habits, sun exposure, poor levels of hydration and poor nutrition can further impact on skin integrity.

The skin's natural moisturiser and water barrier come from sebum; as we age, sebum production reduces and the skin becomes drier and/or more prone to moisture damage. Dry skin can lead to itching, cracking, scaling and inflammation, thereby resulting in breaches of the skin through which bacteria can invade, causing skin infection (cellulitis). Excess moisture on the skin can cause excoriation or maceration, which again breaches this protective layer, thereby increasing the risk of cellulitis.

This chapter will focus on the types of products that are available that can enhance the quality and integrity of the skin, thereby going some way to protect it from the effects of day-to-day living.

Moisturisers

Moisturising is the most effective way of substituting the loss and/or reduction of sebum, as it helps in restoring the barrier function of the epidermis. Indeed, moisturisers are an essential part of daily skin care, as they slow the loss of skin moisture through evaporation. They maintain skin suppleness, prevent drying and cracking, while improving the appearance of the skin.

Moisturisers should ideally be applied twice daily after bathing to intact skin and should not be applied between toes or in skin folds, as this increases the risk of fungal infections in these areas. Their application should be in a downward motion in the direction of hair growth in order to reduce the risk of blocking hair follicles. Typically, moisturisers are made up of water and petroleum. Unperfumed and alcohol-free products are most beneficial to avoid skin irritation or reactions.

Ointments, creams and lotions

Ointments: These products are similar to moisturisers, as they produce a protective layer over the skin. Ointments are typically thicker in consistency than moisturisers and are primarily made from water and oils (e.g. lanolin, which can cause skin reactions in some people).

Creams and lotions: These are thinner in consistency than moisturisers and ointments, as they are made primarily from water. As a result, they are less effective at hydrating dry skin, requiring more frequent applications. They are less occlusive than moisturisers and ointments, so are less effective at protecting from the effects of moisture.

Emollients

Emollients are also known as 'moisturisers'. They can be used to wash the skin and can be applied directly to the skin as with other moisturisers (e.g. Dermol range; see Figure 30.1). Emollients are particularly useful in protecting the skin from irritants (e.g. under bandages); they are the preferred moisturiser for people with sensitive skin and for those who have eczema, as they can prevent flare-ups of these conditions (e.g. Epaderm cream; see Figure 30.2). These products can be purchased directly from a pharmacy and are available on prescription.

Steroid creams and ointments

These products differ from emollients and other moisturisers and are intended to be used to clear up flare-ups of skin conditions, such as eczema. These are not intended for regular use unless directed by a physician. The application of these products is through the fingertip unit theory, except in children. Most steroid creams and ointments are used for 3–5 days on the face and 7–14 days on the body.

Barrier creams

While the aforementioned products (with the exception of steroid creams and ointments) provide an element of moisture blocking, it is advisable to use specific barrier creams (Figure 30.3) on body parts where excess moisture exists. These products have the added benefit of petroleum and/or zinc oxide, which provide a greater degree of moisture blocking. Barrier creams should only be applied to intact skin.

Some barrier creams contain alcohol, which if applied to broken skin causes stinging; such products should be avoided. Similarly, barrier creams that have a thicker consistency cause excess friction on the skin during application and removal; such products should also be avoided as far as possible. Furthermore, these thicker creams are often contraindicated by incontinence pad manufacturers, as they leave a film on the pad that can inhibit their absorbency ability, causing moisture to run off the pad and/or spread to wider areas of unprotected skin. These types of creams also obscure the skin, making observation of the skin difficult.

Barrier sprays

Barrier sprays (Figure 30.3) are useful for use on superficial skin breaks and rashes, for example, on continence lesions, rashes and on peri-wound skin, taking care to avoid the wound itself. Sprays allow adhesive dressings to be applied to the skin, whereas barrier creams do not.

It is essential that products be chosen based on a holistic assessment, and that manufacturer recommendations are always adhered to. Adverse effects of emollients can include stinging and discomfort on dry broken skin, allergic reaction or sensitivity to the preservatives used in some products, folliculitis, reduction of heat loss from the skin in warm weather, fire risk with paraffin-based products, tachyphylaxis (diminishing response to the emollient, cream and spray), slipping in the bath and shower, cross-contamination if surfaces are not kept clean, tubs and tubes left open, and poor concordance when the patient only applies a small amount or stops using the treatment.

31 Advanced technologies

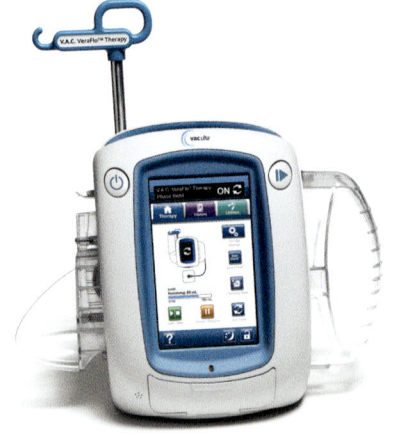

Figure 31.1 VAC pump.

Source: KCI. Used with permission. Courtesy of KCI.

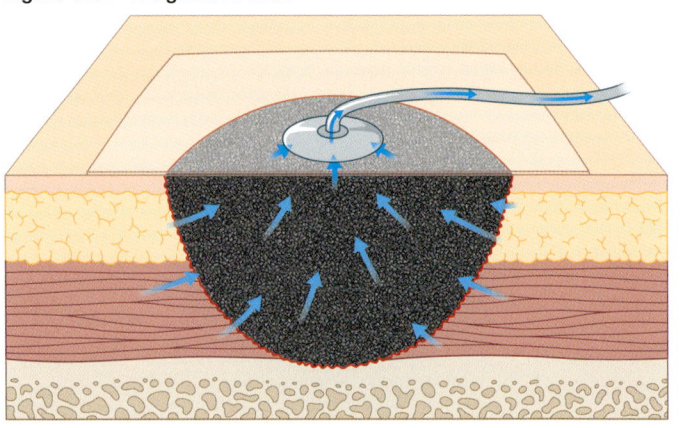

Figure 31.2 Diagram of TNP.

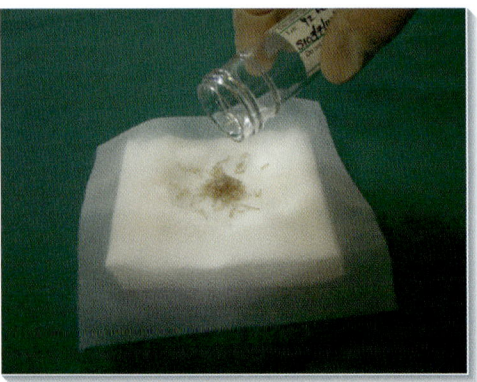

Figure 31.3 Larval therapy.

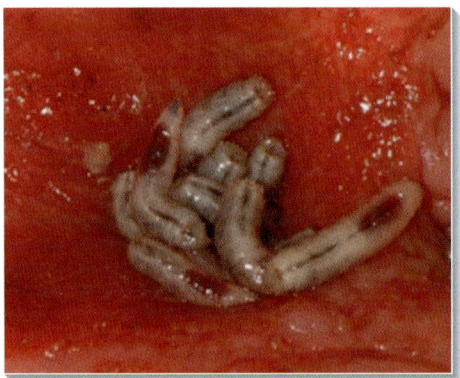

Figure 31.4 Maggots on the wound.

Source: The Surgical Materials Testing Laboratory. Reproduced with permission of The Surgical Materials Testing Laboratory.

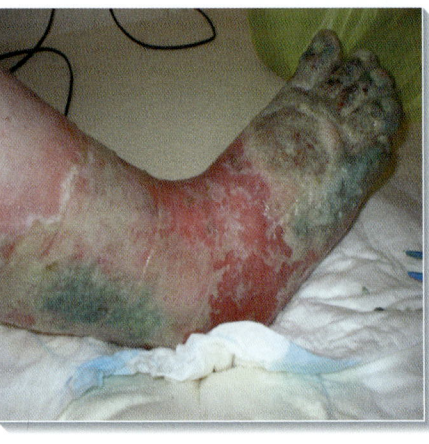

Figure 31.5 Colonies of *Pseudomonas* after larval therapy.

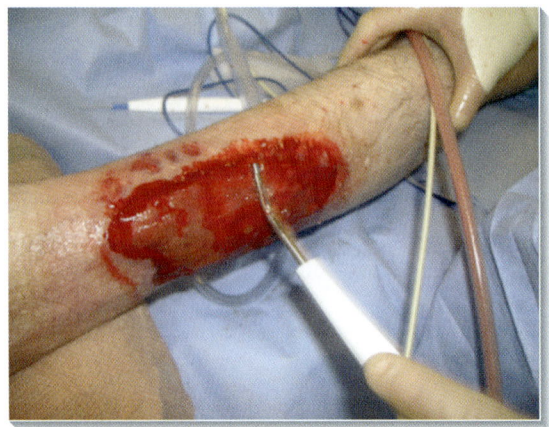

Figure 31.6 Versajet.

Wound Care at a Glance, Second Edition. Ian Peate and Melanie Stephens.
© 2020 John Wiley & Sons Ltd. Published 2020 by John Wiley & Sons Ltd.
Companion website: http://www.ataglanceseries.com/nursing/woundcare/

Research into wound-healing is progressing at significant rates, and much of the work is focused around removing debris and speeding up the healing process of wounds. Additionally, scientists strive to find new ways of preventing infections; however, in some cases, ancient tried-and-tested methods do not appear to have been effectively surpassed to date.

This chapter is intended to give an overview of some of the technologies that are now well established and even ancient, and those that are up and coming, which may or may not be more commonly used in the future.

Topical negative pressure (TNP)

This commonly used technique is also known as 'vacuum-assisted closure' (VAC) therapy; it is where a special dressing type is applied directly to a wound that is sealed in place with a film dressing, which is then attached by tubing to a special suction pump (Figure 31.1). When the pump is operational, it creates suction in the wound, causing negative pressure (Figure 31.2). Negative pressures at 125 mmHg appear to enhance the phases of wound-healing, not least because it increases the blood supply to the wound bed, while providing good exudate control and a moist wound-healing environment. Wounds treated with TNP appear to have fewer complications and have significantly faster healing rates. If the wound is likely to require long-term dressings, TNP can be more cost-effective than traditional dressings over a longer period of time. As dressings only require changing over 48 or 72 hours, this method of wound treatment can reduce nursing time, leaving the patient with greater independence, as this treatment can be suitable for patients in any setting, including in the community.

There are, however, disadvantages with this treatment, including having to fully debride a wound before the treatment can be commenced. This in itself can be time-consuming and costly, so the prevention of debris on a wound with good exudate management is vital to speed up the application of this therapy. Many patients report pain on dressing changes with TNP, making this treatment intolerable, particularly for those with vascular disease in their lower limbs, which is unfortunate as these wounds would benefit from the treatment due to an increased blood flow. The treatment is contraindicated for bleeding wounds, fistulas (unless approved by a specialist) and malignant wounds and any underlying osteomyelitis (bone infection) must be treated for at least 2 weeks prior to the application of this treatment. Other disadvantages of the treatment besides cost are mechanical failures, such as kinked tubing, loss of suction and the inability to achieve a good seal in the first place, especially if the wound is sited near an orifice, such as the anus.

Larval (maggot) therapy

Maggots have been working their magic on wounds for centuries, saving many a life during wartimes. They work by excreting an enzyme that then liquefies dead and devitalised tissues on a wound (Figures 31.3 and 31.4). The maggot then drinks this liquid, thereby removing slough and necrosis from the wound bed, until it eventually reveals healthy granulation tissues. An entire limb can be removed this way if it no longer consists of living tissues. Maggots are, however, contraindicated on fistula wounds and bleeding wounds.

Known affectionately as 'the world's smallest surgeon', maggots will debride a wound faster than autolytic debridement (i.e. using dressings to mimic what maggots do). Interestingly, they are known to eradicate in their gut the bacteria they take in with the wound exudate, including bacteria, such as methicillin-resistant *Staphylococcus aureus* (MRSA). However, *Pseudomonas* appears to upset the maggots, often killing them in large numbers, so they tend to avoid taking in this bacterium. (Figure 31.5 shows a limb after one treatment of larval therapy. The limb was originally covered in slough, much of which was removed by the first treatment. The two 'blue' areas are colonies of *Pseudomonas*, which the maggots did not touch.).

Versajet

This is a device similar to a high-pressure washer; it sprays sterile water at high speed onto the wound in order to evacuate and/or excise debris, bacteria and contaminants from the wound bed (Figure 31.6).

Electrical stimulation

During the process of wound-healing, the body has a system whereby a bioelectrical current is sent to the injured site, which enhances the healing rate of a wound (or any other traumatised tissue or bone). In some cases, this electric current has a short circuit for some reason, and the wound either fails to heal or is very slow to heal.

One of the most exciting developments in wound treatments in recent years is the use of electrostimulation in the non-healing or stagnant wound. It is thought that an external electrical current applied to the wound bed (situated within a dressing) mimics the natural bioelectric current that appears to be absent in the non-healing wound, thereby progressing the wound through the tissue-repair processes mentioned earlier in this book. This treatment then accelerates the healing rate of the wound by attracting neutrophils, increasing the growth of fibroblasts and other growth factors, promoting granulation tissue by increasing the blood flow to the wound bed and finally by inducing epidermal cell migration. Studies have shown significantly improved healing rates on otherwise non-healing wounds when this treatment has been applied.

Interestingly, electrostimulation is thought to attract macrophages to the wound bed, which reduces the risk of infection in these types of wounds. This in itself is a significant breakthrough and would hopefully go some way to boost an individual's immunity, even in wounds that have little prospect of healing due to a significantly reduced blood supply, for example. However, while this treatment shows promise, much more research is needed in the field of electrostimulation before it becomes a treatment choice in chronic, non-healing wounds.

Cell-based and tissue-based therapies

Cellular and tissue-based therapies contain several mixtures of cellular and acellular components meant to stimulate wound-healing and lead to wound closure. The products stimulate or replace the extra cellular matrix and when placed in the wound bed provide a temporary scaffold or support cells to migrate and proliferate to aid wound-healing. The products contain either living cells (cellular) or are inert (acellular), and are sourced from biological tissue (animal, human or plant), synthetic materials or composite materials (biological and synthetic). Products may be classified as biological dressings, skin substitutes, xenografts, allografts or collagen dressings.

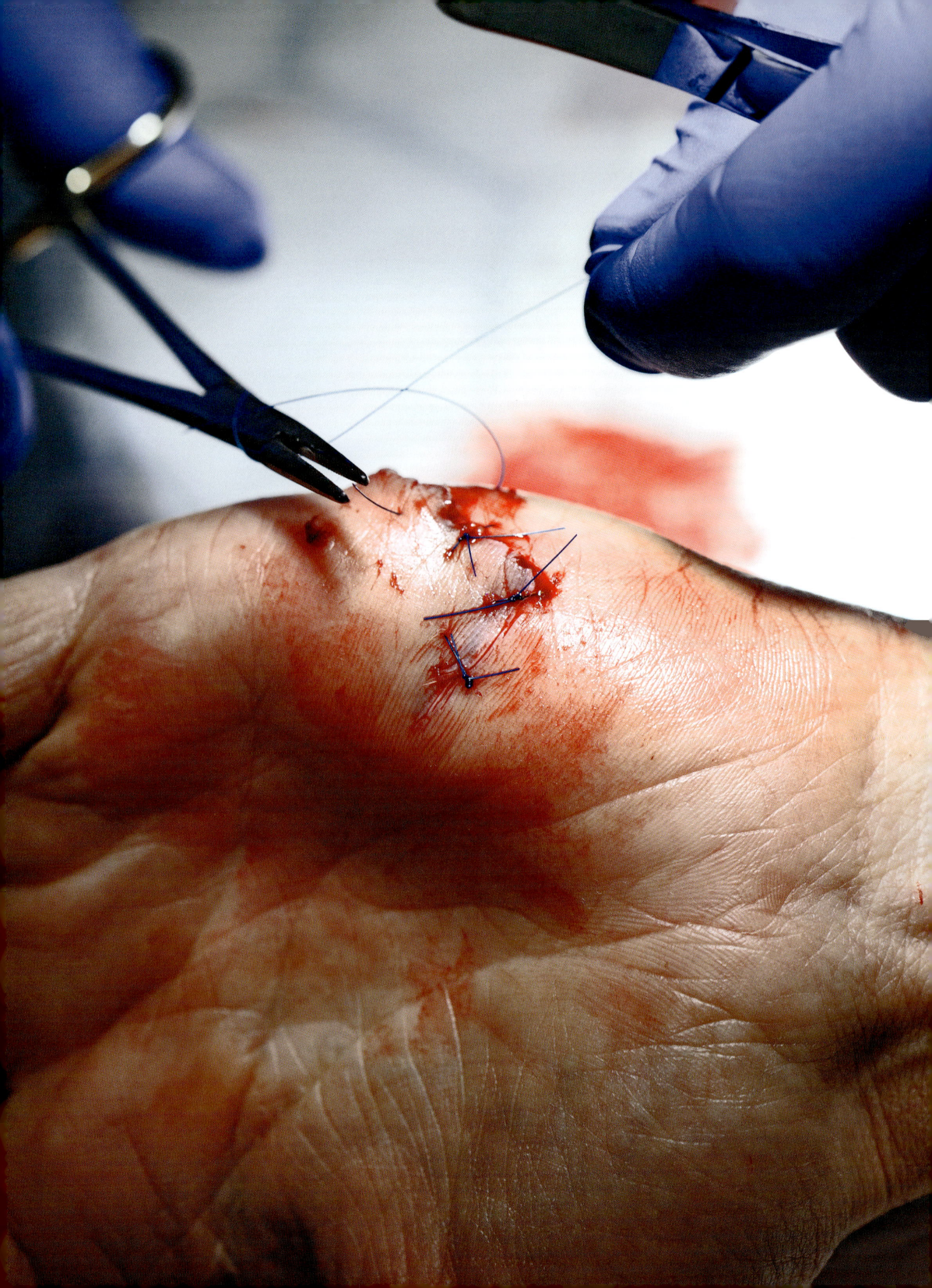

Complexities of wound care

Part 6

Chapters

32	Pressure redistribution equipment	80
33	Pressure ulcer classification and prevention	82
34	Pressure ulcers	86
35	Venous leg ulcers	88
36	Lymphoedema	90
37	Compression therapy	92
38	Arterial ulcers	94
39	Assessing for arterial disease: ankle–brachial pressure index and toe–brachial pressure index	96
40	Interpreting ABPIs	100
41	Diabetic foot ulcers	102
42	Moisture lesions	106
43	Surgical wounds	108
44	Traumatic wounds	112
45	Burns and scalds	114
46	Atypical wounds	116
47	Wounds in different populations	118
48	Malignant wounds and palliative wound care	120

 Visit the companion website at **www.ataglanceseries.com/nursing/woundcare** to test yourself on these topics.

32 Pressure redistribution equipment

Figure 32.1 A static foam mattress.

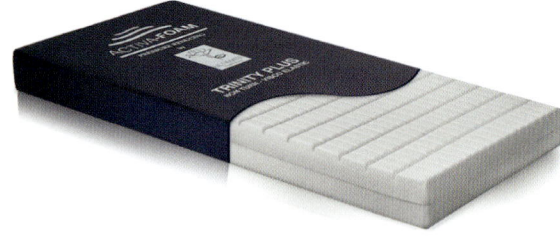

Source: Ultimate Healthcare, Frontier Medical Group. Reproduced with permission of Carl May and Steve Tetlow, Ultimate Healthcare Group.

Figure 32.2 A static pressure-redistributing cushion (foam).

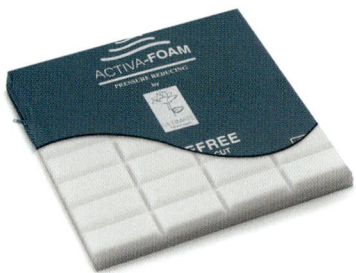

Source: Ultimate Healthcare, Frontier Medical Group. Reproduced with permission of Carl May and Steve Tetlow, Ultimate Healthcare Group.

Figure 32.3 A dynamic alternating air mattress (full replacement).

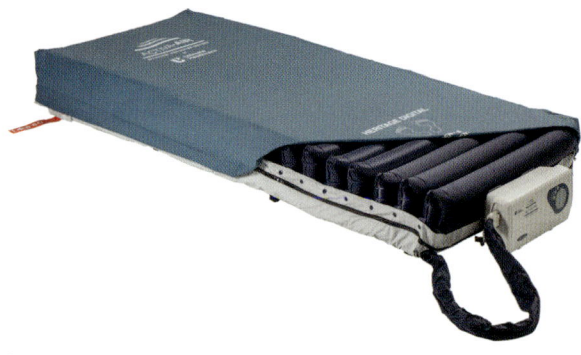

Source: Ultimate Healthcare, Frontier Medical Group. Reproduced with permission of Carl May and Steve Tetlow, Ultimate Healthcare Group.

Figure 32.4 A dynamic alternating air mattress (overlay).

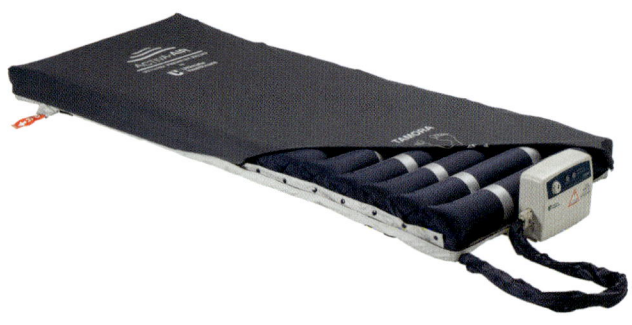

Source: Ultimate Healthcare, Frontier Medical Group. Reproduced with permission of Carl May and Steve Tetlow, Ultimate Healthcare Group.

Figure 32.5 A dynamic alternating air cushion.

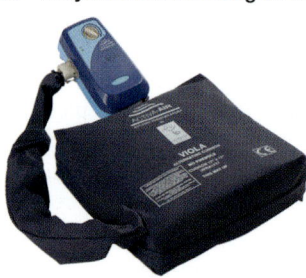

Source: Ultimate Healthcare, Frontier Medical Group. Reproduced with permission of Carl May and Steve Tetlow, Ultimate Healthcare Group.

Figure 32.6 (a) Foot protectors, and (b) supporting wedge.

(a) 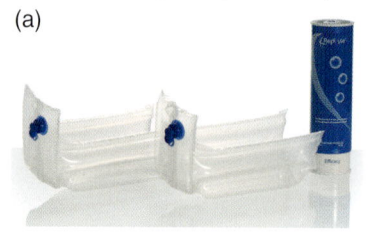   (b)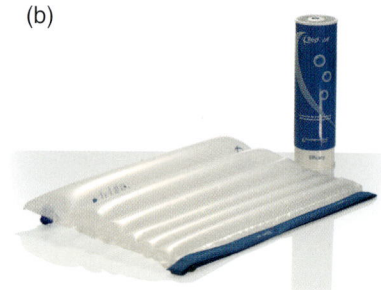

Source: Repose, Frontier Medical Group. Reproduced with permission of Matthew Clutterbuck, Frontier Medical Group.

Wound Care at a Glance, Second Edition. Ian Peate and Melanie Stephens.
© 2020 John Wiley & Sons Ltd. Published 2020 by John Wiley & Sons Ltd.
Companion website: http://www.ataglanceseries.com/nursing/woundcare/

Pressure damage is caused first and foremost by prolonged, unrelieved pressure against the skin and underlying tissues. Pressure damage is exacerbated by the presence of friction and shearing, which makes the skin and underlying tissues more vulnerable to the effects of pressure. The speed at which a pressure ulcer develops depends on many factors that are direct and indirect forces to the patient and these must be addressed as far as possible in order to reduce the probability of developing a pressure ulcer.

The use of appropriate pressure-redistributing devices is one way to deal with extrinsic factors that affect the probability of the patient developing a pressure ulcer. These devices distribute pressure over a greater area, which means pressure ulcers take longer to develop than they otherwise do, if the patient is not nursed on an appropriate pressure-redistributing device.

Therefore, it is very important to point out that patients who are nursed on these devices inevitably develop a pressure ulcer, eventually, if they are not repositioned at regular intervals, regardless of how high the specification of such devices are. These devices simply distribute pressure so that the patient can go for longer without being moved. The frequency of repositioning has been addressed elsewhere in this book.

There is a huge range of products in the market that claim to distribute pressure effectively and the costs of such devices vary widely. Selecting a device depends on the findings of the clinical judgement and on the findings of a pressure ulcer risk assessment. This chapter will give an overview of the main types of devices available and will then discuss their appropriateness based on national guidelines.

National guidelines

NHS Improvement (2018), the Tissue Viability Society (2017), the European Pressure Ulcer Advisory Panel, National Pressure Ulcer Advisory Panel and Pan Pacific Pressure Injury Alliance (2014) and National Institute for Health Care and Clinical Excellent (2014) recommend the following devices to be used for those individuals who are at risk of pressure damage.

1. Any patient who has a Category 3 or 4 pressure ulcer must be nursed on a dynamic air mattress and cushion.
2. Any patient deemed to be at an elevated risk must be nursed on a high-specification (e.g. viscoelastic) foam mattress and cushion, provided he/she has no pressure ulcers greater than Category 2.
3. A standard foam mattress and cushion are suitable for patients who are at risk, who have no pressure ulcers and who can reposition themselves competently and independently.

Determining the level of risk must include the use of a risk assessment tool and clinical judgement, as the risk score may not reflect the clinical findings.

Pressure redistribution devices

Static foam mattresses and cushions

These are available in a variety of sizes that fit most beds and chairs (Figures 32.1 and 32.2). The standard foam mattress/cushion will mean that less pressure distribution is provided, so the patient will require more frequent repositioning than if a high-specification (viscoelastic) foam mattress/cushion was used. These mattresses are also available in bariatric sizes that can accommodate heavier patients. It is therefore important that the patient is weighed regularly to ensure that the most appropriate device is being used.

Dynamic air devices (mattresses and cushions)

These devices are called 'dynamic' due to their active ability to alternate pressure from one area of the body to another, usually by deflating the alternate or every third cell. They can be purchased as either a full replacement mattress (Figure 32.3), as an overlay that lies over a standard or high-specification mattress (Figure 32.4) or as cushions (Figure 32.5). There is little evidence that one type is more effective than the other. The overlay however increases the overall height of the bed as compared to a replacement mattress and is an important consideration if bed rails are required to prevent a patient from rolling out of bed; in such case, a full replacement mattress must be selected. These devices have weight limitations, which vary from one manufacturer to another, so it is important to monitor the patient's weight to ensure they are being nursed on an appropriate device. If a patient requiring a dynamic device is above the highest limit, then a bariatric dynamic device must be selected. If the patient is below the lowest limit, then a low-air-loss mattress must be selected (more information on this mattress type is provided in the following text).

Manufacturer's instructions must be adhered to, and it is usually recommended that nothing other than a loose-fitting sheet and/or the patient's clothing come between the patient and the mattress/cushion, as this negates the efficacy of the dynamics (e.g. if an incontinence sheet is placed under the patient, it is anchored on the inflated cells, which then create a bridge over the deflated cell; the incontinence sheet then presses against the patient's skin, potentially causing pressure damage). This therefore brings into question the need for other devices, such as pillows to elevate heels for example.

Low-air-loss devices

These devices have the same indications as alternating devices, and bariatric versions are available. They are commonly used for low-weight patients who have insufficient weight to 'mould' into the dynamic cells. This type of device is also beneficial to those patients who experience motion sickness from the movement of dynamic cells, and for those who experience pain with this movement. For this reason, they are often the product of choice for the terminally ill.

Tilt-in-space wheelchairs and chairs

For people at risk of developing pressure ulcers, tilt-in-space wheelchairs and chairs are sometimes helpful. In these pieces of equipment, the seat and backrest angles remain fixed, as they are tilted backwards with the occupant staying in the same posture as the seat and back tilt.

Other commonly used devices

There is a range of other devices available that claim to relieve pressure, such as heel protectors and wedges (Figure 32.6), but care/nursing staff must not forget that these devices continue to place pressure against the patient's skin, and so must not be relied upon to fully relieve pressure. Regular skin checks must be carried out to ensure that their continued use remains appropriate.

33 Pressure ulcer classification and prevention

Figure 33.1 Category I pressure ulcer.

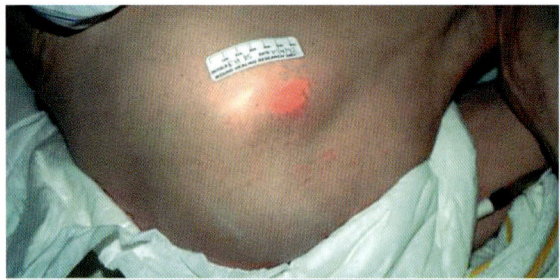

Figure 33.2 Category II pressure ulcer.

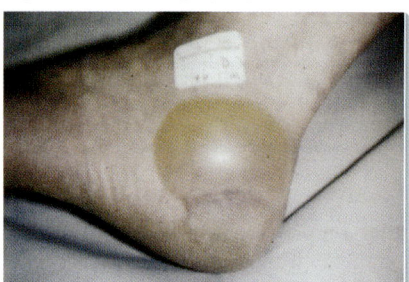

Source: Grey et al 2006, figure 5, p 473. Reproduced with permission of the BMJ.

Figure 33.3 Category III pressure ulcer.

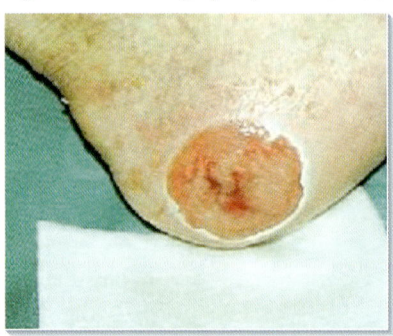

Figure 33.4 Category IV pressure ulcer.

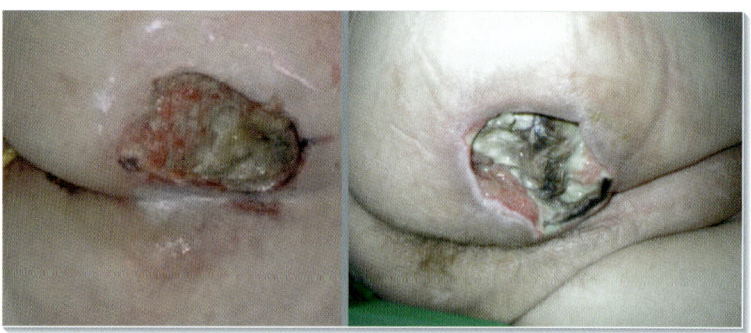

Figure 33.5 Unstageable.

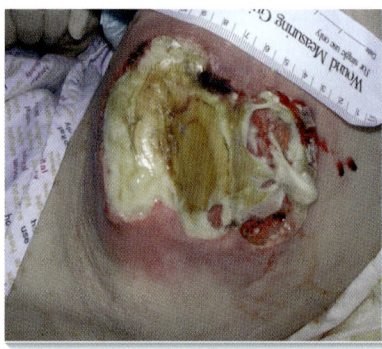

Figure 33.6 Suspected deep tissue injury.

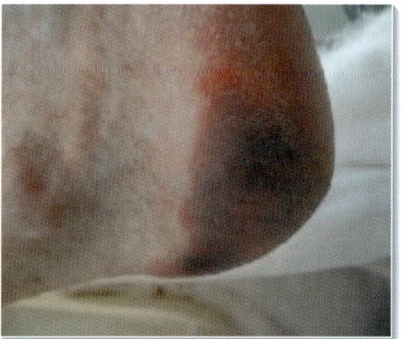

Figure 33.7 Moisture lesion.

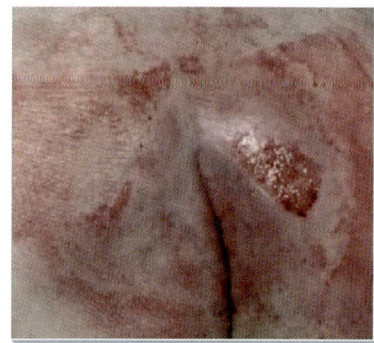

Wound Care at a Glance, Second Edition. Ian Peate and Melanie Stephens.
© 2020 John Wiley & Sons Ltd. Published 2020 by John Wiley & Sons Ltd.
Companion website: http://www.ataglanceseries.com/nursing/woundcare/

Classification of pressure ulcers

Pressure ulcers are classified in the UK using the NNPUAP/EPUAP/PPPIA severity scale, which uses a scale of I to IV, with Category IV being the most severe pressure ulcer.

The definition of each category is as follows:

- *Category I* (Figure 33.1): Intact skin with non-blanchable redness of a localised area usually over a bony prominence. Dark pigmented skin may not have visible blanching; its colour may differ from the surrounding area. The area may be painful, firm, soft, warmer or cooler as compared to adjacent tissues. Category/Stage I may be difficult to detect in individuals with dark skin tones. May indicate 'at risk' individuals (a heralding sign of risk).
- *Category II* (Figure 33.2): Partial-thickness loss of dermis presenting as a shallow open ulcer with a red pink wound bed, without slough. May also present as an intact or open/ruptured serum-filled blister. Presents as a shiny or dry shallow ulcer without slough or bruising. This category/stage should not be used to describe skin tears, tape burns, perineal dermatitis, maceration or excoriation. Bruising indicates suspected deep tissue injury
- *Category III* (Figure 33.3): Full-thickness tissue loss. Subcutaneous fat may be visible but bone, tendon or muscle are not exposed. Slough may be present but does not obscure the depth of tissue loss. May include undermining and tunnelling. The depth of a Category/Stage III pressure ulcer varies by anatomical location. The bridge of the nose, ear, occiput and malleolus do not have subcutaneous tissues, and Category/Stage III ulcers can be shallow. By contrast, areas of significant adiposity can develop extremely deep Category/Stage III pressure ulcers. Bone/tendon is not visible or directly palpable.
- *Category/Stage IV* (Figure 33.4): Full-thickness tissue loss with exposed bone, tendon or muscle. Slough or eschar may be present on some parts of the wound bed. Often includes undermining and tunnelling. The depth of a Category/Stage IV pressure ulcer varies by anatomical location. The bridge of the nose, ear, occiput and malleolus do not have subcutaneous tissues and these ulcers can be shallow. Category/Stage IV ulcers can extend into muscle and/or supporting structures (e.g., fascia, tendon or joint capsule), making osteomyelitis possible. Exposed bone/tendon is visible or directly palpable.

In 2018, a task and finish group were asked by NHS Improvement to review the current classification and measurement of pressure ulcers nationally in England. As a consequence, two categories, *unstageable* and *deep tissue injury*, were added to recommendations for organisations to follow.

- *Unstageable* (Figure 33.5): Full-thickness tissue loss in which the base of the ulcer is covered by slough (yellow, tan, grey, green or brown) and/or eschar (tan, brown or black) in the wound bed. Until enough slough and/or eschar is removed to expose the base of the wound, the true depth and therefore the category/stage, cannot be determined. Stable (dry, adherent and intact without erythema or fluctuance) eschar on the heels serves as 'the body's natural (biological) cover' and should not be removed.
- *Suspected deep tissue injury – depth unknown* (Figure 33.6): Purple or maroon localised area of discoloured intact skin or blood-filled blister due to damage of underlying soft tissues from pressure and/or shear. The area may be preceded by tissues that are painful, firm, mushy, boggy, warmer or cooler as compared to adjacent tissues. Deep tissue injury may be difficult to detect in individuals with dark skin tones. Evolution may include a thin blister over a dark wound bed. The wound may further evolve and become covered by thin eschar. Evolution may be rapid, exposing additional layers of tissues even with optimal treatment.
- *Moisture lesions* (Figure 33.7): These are not pressure ulcers, but wounds that are caused by prolonged contact with moisture. These are often incorrectly categorised as Grade II ulcers due to the dermal loss that occurs with maceration and/or excoriation. This damage can however increase the speed at which a pressure ulcer develops, if not appropriately managed.

Prevention of pressure ulcers

By April 2019, most NHS trusts should have adopted a model of care known as ASSKING, which, when adopted as SSKIN in patient care, has been shown to reduce the incidence of pressure ulcers. It has also been shown to increase the healing rates of the existing pressure damage.

However, it is important to assess and address all other influencing factors noted on pressure ulcer risk assessment, as well as implementing care in accordance with the following ASSKING care bundle:

- *A = Assess*: Assess risk within 6 hours of admission, which includes the use of an appropriate risk assessment tool, such as Purpose T and Braden.
- *S = Skin*: The skin is observed on admission, and any pressure damage is recorded on a body map.
  - The body map is repeated each time a reassessment of risk is carried out.
  - Additionally, the patient's skin should be observed for signs of pressure damage at each position change, and at least once on every shift.
  - The findings should be recorded on the care plan evaluation.
- *S = Surface*: Following the assessment of risk, the correct pressure relieving devices (e.g. cushions and mattresses) must be installed under the patient.
  - The choice of equipment used is determined by the holistic risk assessment result, and the specific device used must be recorded in the patient's notes (discussed in the following chapter).
- *K = Keep moving*: NICE recommends that no patient be left in the same position for longer than 4 hours (adults at high risk) and 6 hours (adults at risk) when in bed and no longer than 2 hours when sitting in a chair, provided the patient is on adequate pressure-relieving surfaces.
  - Those at greater risk require more frequent repositioning than this, similar to those who are awaiting pressure-relieving surfaces.
  - It is vital that every position change be recorded on a turn/repositioning chart to enable continuity of care and to alert others when repositioning is required.
  - In case of a pressure damage, or if an existing ulcer deteriorates, the frequency of repositioning must be increased without delay following reassessment.
- *I = Incontinence*: This section must not be limited to urine and faecal incontinence, but consideration must also be given to any moisture that may be in contact with the skin for prolonged periods; for example, sweat, wound exudate, or leakage from catheters or stoma bags and drink spillages.
  - Adopting a regular toileting regimen prevents incontinence, whilst providing repositioning and therefore regular pressure relief for the patient.
  - When there is a risk of moisture getting onto the skin, it is essential that good skin care be provided using appropriate wash creams and moisture barriers.

- *N = Nutrition*: As stated in the previous chapter, reduced nutrition is the second highest reason why an individual will develop pressure ulcers.
  - It is therefore vital that a nutrition assessment is completed as soon as possible after admission to the care setting, and diet and fluids are monitored to ensure that adequate nutrients are taken by the patient.
  - NICE recommends the use of the Malnutrition Universal Screening Tool (MUST) on admission and at weekly intervals along with weekly weight measurement (or monthly, if the penitent is cared for by district nurses). Reassessments must be carried out in the event of a patient failing to take sufficient diet and fluids, or if he/she demonstrates any weight loss.
  - In these instances, food supplements must be provided and a referral to a GP or a dietician must be made without delay. Further, if a patient develops a Grade III or IV pressure ulcer, it is also advisable to refer the patient to the dietician due to the need for increased nutrition to aid healing.
- *G = Giving information*: Understanding to communicate effectively with patients, carers and the interprofessional team increases awareness and improves concordance and engagement in pressure ulcer prevention and management strategies.

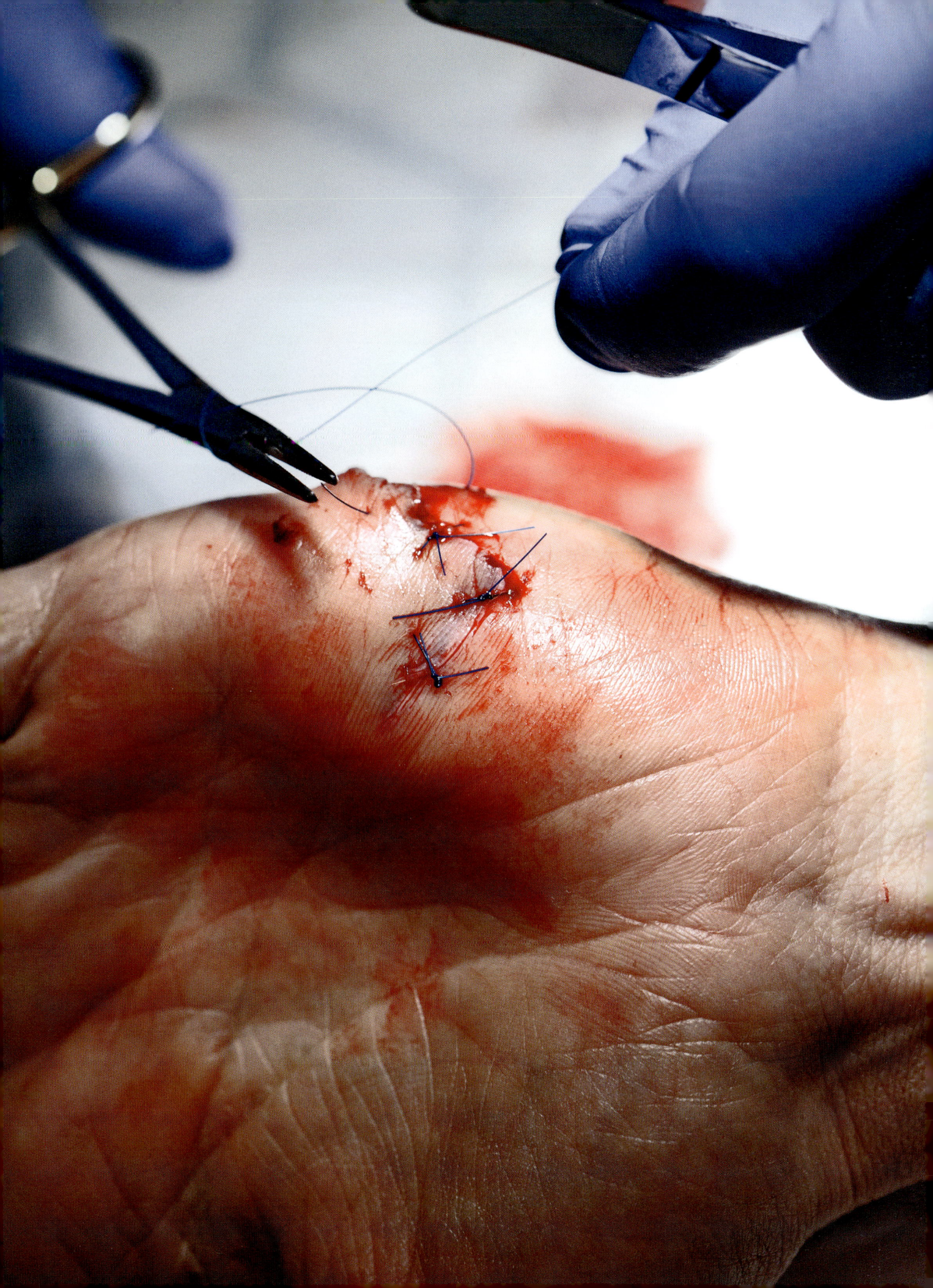

34 Pressure ulcers

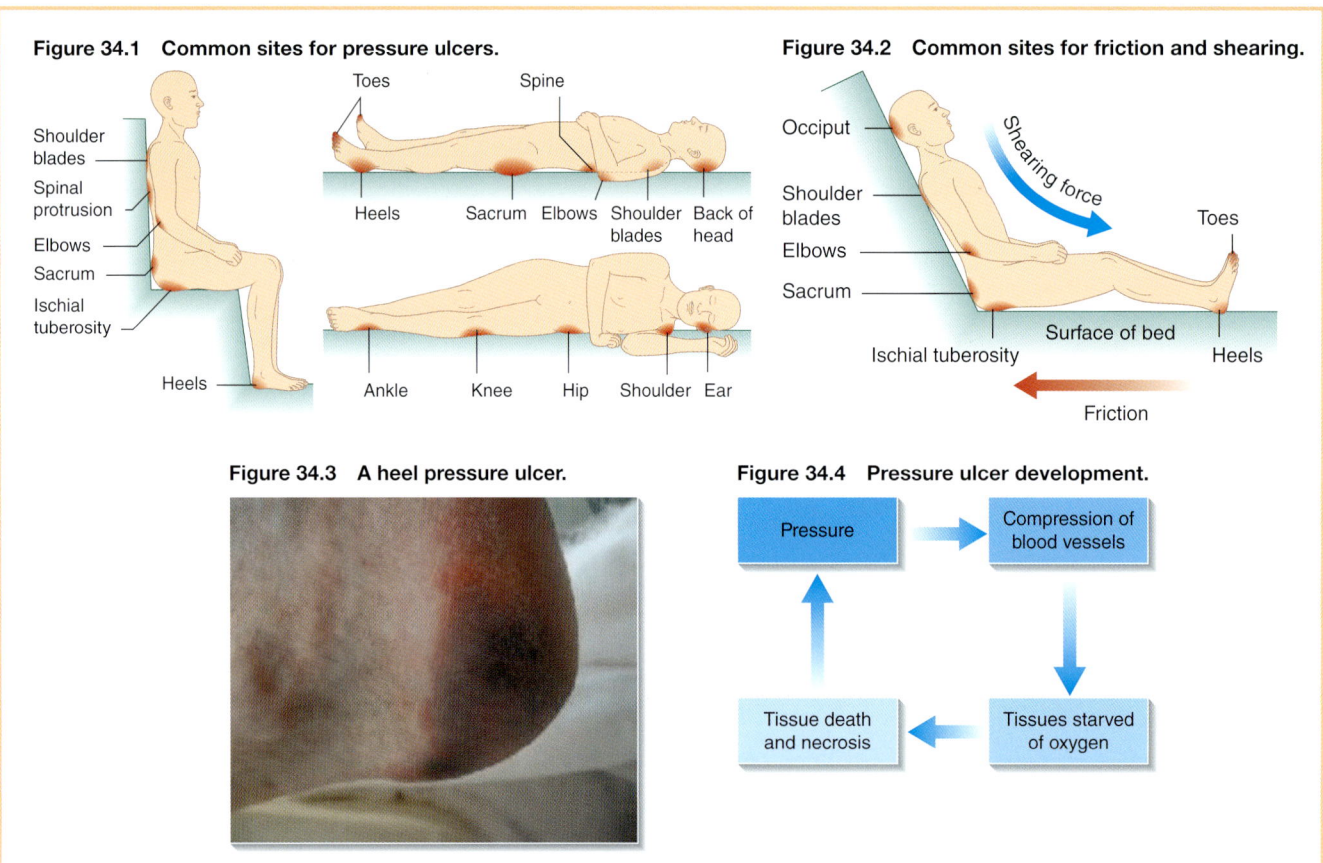

Figure 34.1 Common sites for pressure ulcers.

Figure 34.2 Common sites for friction and shearing.

Figure 34.3 A heel pressure ulcer.

Figure 34.4 Pressure ulcer development.

Wound Care at a Glance, Second Edition. Ian Peate and Melanie Stephens.
© 2020 John Wiley & Sons Ltd. Published 2020 by John Wiley & Sons Ltd.
Companion website: http://www.ataglanceseries.com/nursing/woundcare/

Pressure ulcers are also known as bed sores, pressure sores and pressure damage or decubitus ulcers. They can occur on any part of the body, but are seen most commonly over bony prominences, such as the occiput (back of the head), sacrum, elbows, heels, hips and the ischial tuberosities (the bones we sit on) (Figures 34.1, 34.2 and 34.3). One common pressure ulcer that occurs is on the feet due to rubbing of shoes, although most people do not recognise this as pressure damage. This chapter will deal with the causes and assessment of pressure ulcers and risk. The following chapter will deal with ulcer classification and prevention.

Aetiology

Pressure damage is predominantly caused by prolonged and unrelieved pressure from any external object against the skin (e.g. bed, chair, clothing, footwear, medical devices, etc.). The applied pressure occludes blood vessels (capillaries and venules) in the skin and underlying tissues, which means that there is insufficient or no blood supply to the affected tissues that then die due to lack of oxygen (ischaemia); further, there is a formation of waste products due to the occlusion of venules, which causes reduced tissue viability leading to poor tissue repair (Figure 34.4). It is similar to a boulder being placed on a hose pipe that feeds a garden; failure to remove the boulder to allow water through results in the garden drying up and dying. Patients who are immobile or have difficulty responding independently to pressure, or those who have a neurological deficit and cannot feel the effects of pressure, are at immediate risk of developing pressure damage.

Additional causes

There are many factors that affect an individual's likelihood of developing pressure ulcers – the more factors involved, the greater the risk score is, and the faster a pressure ulcer is likely to develop. It is therefore essential to carry out a risk assessment that considers all potential contributory factors, so that an appropriate level of care can be planned and implemented. Here, some of the main factors are considered:

- *Friction*: The regular rubbing of the skin removes the epithelial cells, and, if not protected, damages the cuboidal cells, causing a breach to the skin, through which bacteria can enter. If pressure is applied to this area also, then a pressure ulcer develops faster than it would otherwise do (Figure 34.2).
- *Shearing*: Happens when two types of tissues are forced in opposite directions, causing tearing and inflammation at the site of trauma, usually deep within the tissues and commonly at the site of underlying bones. If pressure is applied to the area, a pressure ulcer develops faster than it would otherwise do if shearing had not occurred (Figure 34.2).
- *Incontinence, moisture and sweating*: Moisture that is in constant or regular contact with the skin causes maceration (i.e. water logging) or excoriation (i.e. burning), which makes the skin much more vulnerable to pressure. Skin damage from moisture gives the pressure damage a head start.
- *Poor nutrition*: After immobility, reduced nutritional intake is the next main cause of pressure damage; poor nutrition leads to lethargy, reduced mobility, reduced cell regeneration and poor healing rates. It is therefore essential that the patient be encouraged to take adequate nutrition and fluids in order to reduce the risk of developing pressure ulcers, and to improve healing rates in cases where they exist. The recommended daily intake for a male is around 2000 kcal, and for females it is around 1600 kcal per day. These calories are required for daily activities and normal cell regeneration. If a wound exists, the patient requires a higher intake of nutrients, particularly of protein, in order to improve wound-healing rates.
- *Underlying comorbidities*: There are many medical conditions that make an individual more likely to develop pressure damage as compared to the risk level of a healthy individual. For example, diabetes, peripheral vascular disease, other vascular diseases (e.g. vascular dementia) and coronary artery disease have an effect on the circulation, and can affect the circulation of blood to the skin also. When pressure is applied, the (probably) already reduced blood supply is reduced even further, making pressure damage occur more quickly. In conditions such as malignancy, organ failure or in general malaise, the catabolic rate (i.e. tissue breakdown rate) is faster than in a healthy individual, which means that there is a need for increased nutrition, yet these patients usually do not feel like eating, keeping them at very high risk of developing pressure damage.
- *Medications*: Certain medications are known to impact on the tissue viability of a patient; for example, steroids and cytotoxic drugs, and these patients are at increased risk of developing pressure ulcers if they are not regularly moving or repositioning.

Risk assessment

The National Health Service (NHS) Improvement (2018) and the National Institute for Health and Care Excellence (NICE 2015) recommend that all patients be assessed for risk of pressure ulceration within 6 hours of admission to any care setting (within 24 hours on a district nurse case load). Reassessments must be carried out at least weekly (monthly on a district nurse case load), but sooner in the event the patient's condition changes, if pressure ulcers commence or if existing pressure ulcer deteriorates. Although these time frames are not specifically mentioned in the 2014 guidelines, a responsible body of nurses continues to adhere to this standard.

However, NICE warns that risk assessment tools must be used with caution and should only be used as an aide-memoire only, and to evidence that an assessment has taken place. This is because, for example, a patient who is completely immobile but free from any other risk factors (with a zero risk score) is automatically at risk, whereas a patient with a very high risk score who is fully mobile and able to respond independently to pressure is at no risk. In the event that this patient becomes immobile, then he/she develops a pressure ulcer faster than the immobile patient with a low or zero risk score.

A word of warning: The patients often overlooked as being at no risk are those living with dementia and/or learning disabilities, as they are often very mobile. However, these patients, although fully mobile, are at an elevated risk due to their inability to respond to the effects of pressure (e.g. the feeling of numbness while sitting for too long).

A study funded by the National Institute for Health Research, however, sought to develop and evaluate a new pressure ulcer assessment tool, called PURPOSE-T. This tool assesses eight risk factors: mobility; skin; previous pressure ulcer; sensory perception; perfusion (blood flow); nutrition; moisture and diabetes. Testing in clinical practice by nurses showed very good conformity between the tool and assessors. The PURPOSE-T tool has many advantages over the various current assessment tools, which show numerous inconsistencies and are evidence-based. PURPOSE-T is already being used by many trusts and could assist with the treatment of pressure ulcers.

35 Venous leg ulcers

Figure 35.1 Normal venous flow.

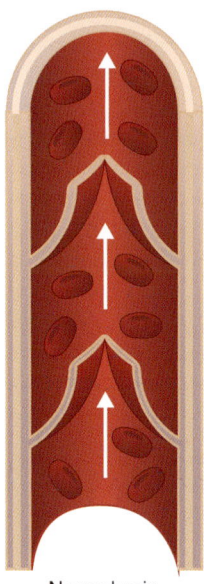

Normal vein

Source: P. Vong. Reproduced with permission of P. Vong.

Figure 35.2 Incompetent venous flow.

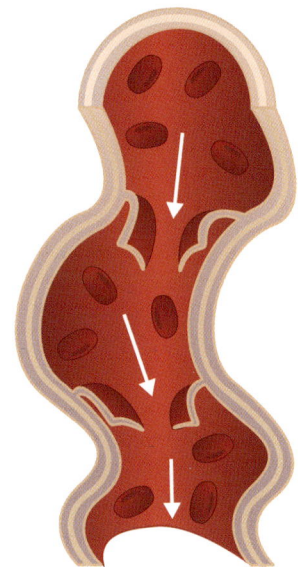

Varicose vein

Source: P. Vong. Reproduced with permission of P. Vong.

Figure 35.3 Venous leg ulcer.

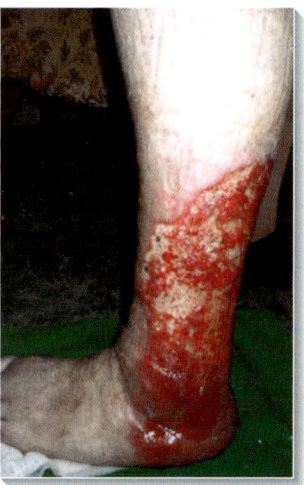 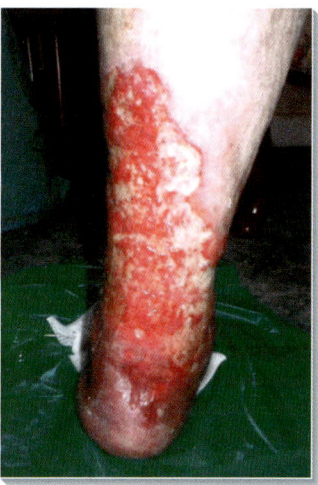 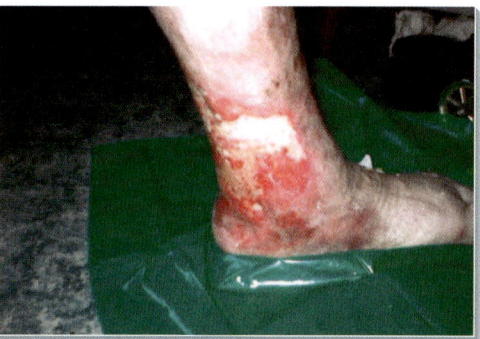

Wound Care at a Glance, Second Edition. Ian Peate and Melanie Stephens.
© 2020 John Wiley & Sons Ltd. Published 2020 by John Wiley & Sons Ltd.
Companion website: http://www.ataglanceseries.com/nursing/woundcare/

Venous insufficiency

Venous leg ulcers occur as a result of venous insufficiency and are thought to affect around 1–2% of the adult population. Venous leg ulcers are accountable for around 70–90% of all leg ulceration in the UK. Fortunately, conservative treatment resolves most venous leg ulcers.

Aetiology

The veins are responsible for carrying deoxygenated blood back to the heart from the tissue capillaries. Venous blood contains high levels of carbon dioxide and metabolic waste collected from the tissues that are disposed of, and the blood is reoxygenated as it flows through the entire circulatory system. The veins help dispose of around 90% of waste fluid, provided there is no incompetence present.

The venous system has three types of veins: deep, superficial and perforating. The deep veins lie within the muscles, are parallel to a neighbouring artery and are responsible for carrying 80–90% of the blood back to the heart. Using the muscles assists with effective venous return by reducing the pressure on the vein walls from the volume of blood within; as the muscles contract, it pushes the blood along the vein towards the heart, thereby reducing the venous pressures. Superficial veins lie within the more superficial tissues and are responsible for draining the skin and subcutaneous tissues. The pressures in these veins are less than in deeper veins. Perforating veins connect the deep and superficial veins throughout the lower leg.

Medium and large veins have bicuspid valves that allow one-directional blood flow (Figure 35.1). However, as blood in the legs flows against gravity, this places undue pressure on the valves, which can then collapse, rendering a valve incompetent (Figure 35.2). When one valve collapses, it places undue pressure on the lower valve, resulting in its collapse as well. As more valves collapse, the entire vein, or parts of the vein, become incompetent. This incompetence then leads to backflow and venous stasis (static blood within the vein), and can lead to varicosities, deep vein thrombosis, phlebitis (inflammation of the vein walls) and/or formation of waste and carbon dioxide in the surrounding tissues. The leakage and/or formation of these waste products in the surrounding tissues can lead to spontaneous development of a leg ulcer, or in the event of trauma, a non-healing wound.

Once a vein becomes incompetent, it is irreparable, and thus venous insufficiency becomes a lifetime condition. On occasions, a vascular surgeon may remove a vein in order to minimise the risk of thrombosis; however, this then places increased pressure on surrounding veins, as the venous return re-routes itself, which increases the risk of further venous incompetence.

Risk factors

Inactivity of the calf muscle is the main cause of venous incompetence and leg ulceration, for example, sitting or standing still for long periods. Other factors are previous venous ulceration, advancing age, trauma, pregnancy, family history, gender (more women than men), obesity, diet, reduced mobility, malnutrition, smoking, diabetes mellitus and drug use.

Symptoms

The symptoms of venous insufficiency can include mild to moderate pain that is relieved on limb elevation; oedema; cellulitis (skin infection); brown staining (pigmentation – lipodermatosclerosis); induration (i.e. woody, lumpy texture of underlying tissues due to the formation of lymph and waste products); itching and less elastic skin than healthy tissues. Healing rates are poor where a wound exists (in undiagnosed ulcers). The ulcer is usually located on the gaiter area of the leg just above the malleolus. The ulcer is usually shallow with sloping edges, and can be extensive in an aspect that may cover the circumference of the gaiter area; there is usually a large amount of wound exudate due to the escape of oedema resulting from the venous incompetence (Figure 35.3). In the absence of arterial disease (discussed later), foot pulses are usually present, and the feet are usually warm to touch and pink in colour.

Diagnosis

As always, diagnosis is made following holistic and clinical assessment. The clinical assessment includes a Doppler ultrasound assessment in order to obtain an ankle–brachial pressure index (ABPI), which confirms or rules out any arterial involvement. This is important, as the treatment for venous insufficiency is usually contraindicated in the presence of arterial insufficiency (discussed in other chapters). A normal ABPI is between 1.0 and 1.2.

Treatment of venous insufficiency

The intervention is aimed at reducing the venous hypertension and providing mechanical support by way of compression hosiery or bandaging to the incompetent veins. Activity that uses the calf muscles must be encouraged, and prolonged sitting or standing must be avoided. Elevation of the legs, so that they are slightly higher than the heart, should be encouraged to ease pressure off the valves and allow gravity to remove the waste products instead. Venous insufficiency means a lifestyle change must be adopted, as it is an incurable condition that means the patient will always be at a risk of leg ulceration and non-healing traumatic wounds.

Treatment of venous ulcers

Good skin care is essential. Hence, on removal of the compression therapy, wash the patient's leg with emollients (using a basin with tap water is adequate), pat the peri-wound skin and leg dry with a clean, soft towel and apply emollients to the skin, avoiding the wound itself and between toes. The most appropriate dressing should be applied following assessment of the wound (see the chapters on wound treatments and dressing choices), and compression therapy must be reapplied. It is common for compression bandages to be used when an ulcer exists due to the difficulties in applying compression hosiery. Once the ulcer heals, compression hosiery can be used on a continuing basis in order to avoid recurrence of the ulcers.

36 Lymphoedema

Figure 36.1 Cavity wound on a lymphoedematous limb treated with larval therapy.

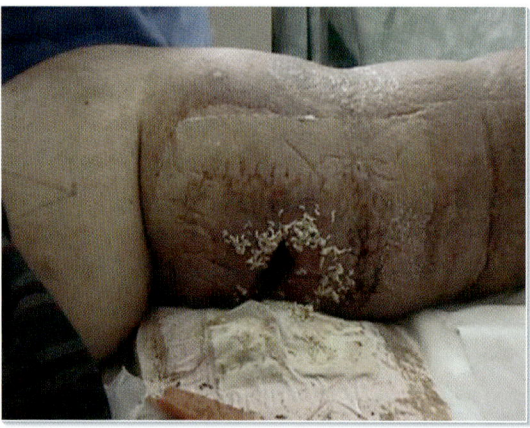

Figure 36.2 Lymphoedema of the left leg. The right leg has chronic oedema.

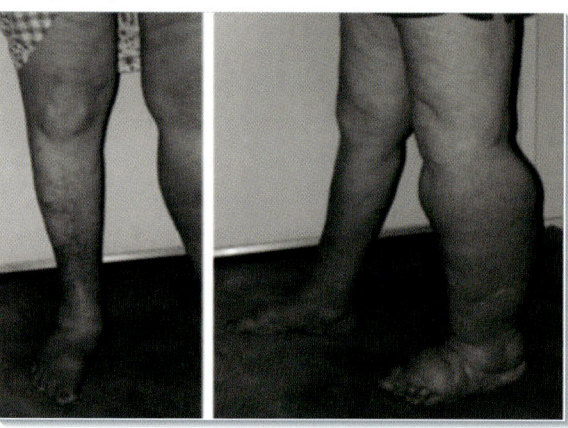

Source: Lawenda et al 2009, figure 8, p. 14. Reproduced with permission of John Wiley & Sons.

Figure 36.3 Lymphoedema of the upper limb following mastectomy and removal of axillary lymph nodes.

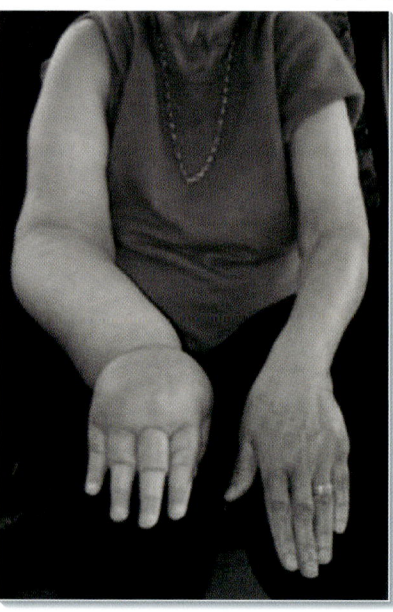

Source: Lawenda et al 2009, Figure 7, p. 14. Reproduced with permission of John Wiley & Sons, Ltd.

Figure 36.4 Unilateral lymphoedema with a healthy right leg.

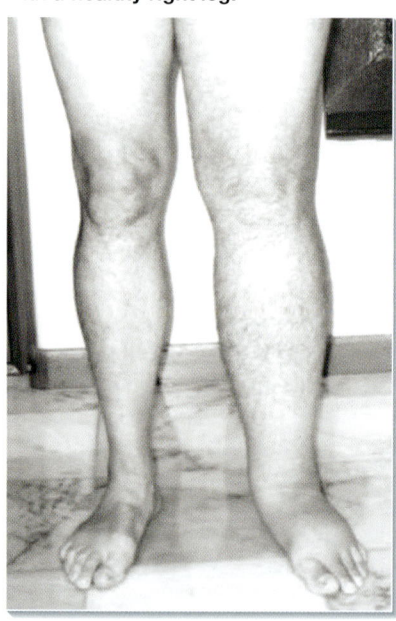

Source: Lawenda et al 2009, Figure 6, p. 13. Reproduced with permission of John Wiley & Sons.

Wound Care at a Glance, Second Edition. Ian Peate and Melanie Stephens.
© 2020 John Wiley & Sons Ltd. Published 2020 by John Wiley & Sons Ltd.
Companion website: http://www.ataglanceseries.com/nursing/woundcare/

The lymphatic system

Lymphoedema is a condition in which there is an accumulation of protein-rich lymph fluid due to a deformation or destruction of lymph nodes, or if there is an impaired transport of lymph around the body. It can affect any part of the body depending on what part of the system or lymph nodes is affected by congenital defect, trauma, surgical removal or disease. The typical onset of primary lymphoedema is at birth and at puberty in males and females and at first pregnancy and the menopause in females. The onset of secondary lymphoedema results from disease (e.g. cancer), trauma and chronic oedema.

The lymphatic system has two main functions: it assists with the regulation of fluid in the body, ridding the body of around 10% of waste fluid per day, absorbing larger molecules than the venous system can deal with. Therefore, together the venous and the lymphatic system remove 100% waste fluids from the body each day; also, it is part of the immune system.

The lymphatic system is part of the circulatory system, and, in effect, it recycles blood plasma around the body. This fluid, known as lymph, travels through a network of vessels similar to the venous and arterial systems. It flows into progressively larger vessels, and is pushed along by skeletal muscle contraction and the respiratory pump towards larger 'collectors' and on to regional lymph nodes. If any part of this system is destroyed or impaired for any reason, the fluid does not reach its destination and gets accumulated in the tissues below the affected vessels, collectors or lymph nodes. Lymph nodes contain lymphoid cells that produce lymphocytes, which assist the body's immune system.

Regional lymph nodes are located in areas, such as the ankle, knee and groin, which remove lymph fluid from the lower limbs into the lower abdomen nodes, and in the wrist, elbow, neck and axilla, which remove lymph from the head and upper limbs into the chest and then the upper abdomen nodes.

When any of these nodes are damaged or diseased, the lymph fluid accumulates in the tissues up to the affected lymph node, causing an increase in size of the affected limb (Figures 36.1–36.4). Elevation of the limb does not allow drainage of this excess fluid, and current treatments are restricted to massage and compression bandaging that force the lymph from the tissues and back towards the lymphatic system for drainage.

The guidance offered by specialist services leads to self-management of the condition and involves four components: sustaining a daily skin care regimen; being as active as feasible; daily application of compression garments and maintaining a healthy weight.

Daily skin care regimen

It is essential that good skin care is encouraged using wash creams and emollients (discussed in Chapter 30), ensuring that the skin and skin folds are fully dried prior to the application of these products. As the limb increases in size, the skin folds require exceptional care to avoid fungal infections, soreness from maceration/sweating and pressure damage from the weight of skin on skin.

Being active

It is known that oedema can be worsened by immobility and gravitational forces; therefore, patients with lymphoedema are encouraged, as much as they can, to be active. Exercise helps lymph move through the lymphatic system from muscle tissue, squeezing the lymph vessels. The assessment of a patient's ability to exercise is necessary, as the lymphoedema specialist ascertains how fit the patient was before treatment started, the type of treatment being provided and how severe the lymphoedema is. Once assessed, the patient is encouraged to start slowly and gently with exercise, progressing gradually to a regular daily routine. This also includes times in the day for leg elevation.

Compression

The compression therapy must only be applied when diagnosis and treatment is confirmed. It must only be applied by a practitioner who has been trained and is competent in the practice of lymphoedema compression bandaging. The pressures used in lymphoedema compression therapy are usually higher than for venous ulceration; in the UK, this is usually at around 50 mmHg pressure.

Prior to the application of compression, careful preparation must be undertaken to applying wadding to the folds, in order to protect from pressure and to ensure the limb is structured into a cylindrical shape. The compression is then applied from the tip of each individual toe, along the foot and up to the groin. As the lymph fluid is squeezed into the major lymph node in the groin for disposal, the limb is gradually reduced in size. The bandages then need to be removed and immediately reapplied to further reduce the lymph and size of the limb. This process must be followed until the limb is reduced to an acceptable size; compression must be continually applied thereafter in order to prevent the formation of lymph in the limb again.

When the upper limb is affected, care must be taken to ensure that rings are not tight; it is advisable to remove rings, as the size of the limb inevitably increases without treatment and could therefore hinder the arterial supply to the fingers. Pressure garments must also be fit for purpose, so that the patient can apply and remove the garments daily. If dexterity and mobility affect the daily application and removal of pressure garments, aids and social care can also be accessed.

Wound management

The primary treatment is to deal with the underlying cause of the lymphoedema and this should entail a referral to a specialist centre so that an accurate diagnosis can be made before commencing treatment. Any failure in managing this condition delays wound healing.

In the meantime, it is important to carry out a holistic assessment in order to identify any influencing factors that could contribute to additional delays in wound healing.

When a wound occurs on a limb affected by lymphoedema, there is an elevated risk of cellulitis and/or wound infection due to the lack of lymph drainage and reduced immunity due to ineffective lymphatics. It is therefore vital that wounds are avoided as far as possible by the provision of good skin care and by avoiding using the affected limb for venepuncture or cannulation.

The principles of wound healing and treatments apply in most cases, as discussed in other chapters.

Maintaining a healthy weight

When a patient is overweight, he/she stores more adipose tissues. This creates a higher volume of blood and lymph in the limbs, placing a greater burden on the ability of lymphatic systems to drain fluid from the tissues. There are many causes of lymphoedema; however, maintaining a healthy weight is necessary to prevent excess strain on joints and muscles too.

Limbs affected by lymphoedema require referral to and a treatment plan by a specialist. In the meantime, it is essential that good skin care be provided, tight-fitting garments and rings removed and only trained and competent clinicians apply compression therapy to the affected limbs. Following holistic assessment, wounds must be treated in accordance with the principles of wound management, as detailed in other chapters.

37 Compression therapy

Figure 37.1 3M Coban 2 compression system bandage.

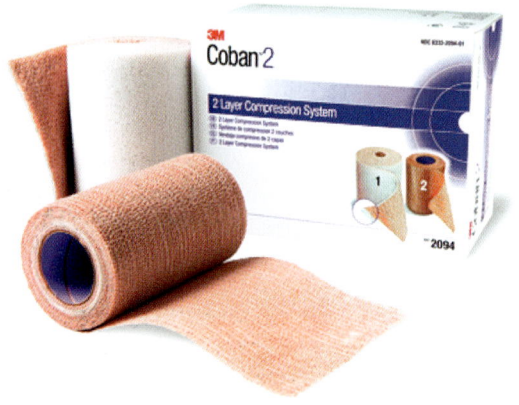

Source: Image © 3M. Reproduced with permission of 3M.

Figure 37.2 Compression hosiery.

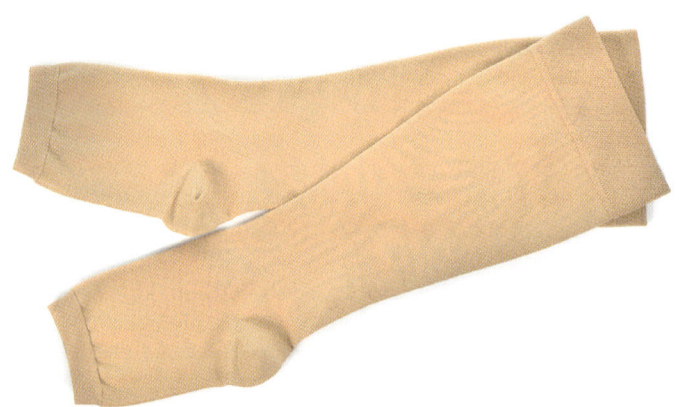

Source: iStock © Geo-grafika.

Box. 37.1 Laplace's law.

$$\text{Bandage compression} = \frac{\text{Tension / layers applied / constant}}{\text{Limb girth / bandage width}}$$

Table 37.1 Selecting the right compression for the patient.

	Bandage system	Leg ulcer hosiery kit	British compression hosiery
Therapy choice	Two-layer or four-layer bandage system normally provides 40 mmHg sustained graduated compression (20 mmHg for reduced compression)	Leg hosiery kit normally provides 40 mmHg ankle (combination of a liner (10 mmHg) and British Standard Class III stockings (30 mmHg))	Class I: 14–17 mmHg at the ankle Class II: 18–24 mmHg at the ankle Class III: 24–35 mmHg at the ankle British Standard Hosiery
Patient assessment	Consider when patient prefers bandages Patient unable to self-manage Regular clinical contact required due to concordance	Consider when patient is non-concordant with bandages Patient must be able to self-manage the application of hosiery Consider if patient prefers the look of hosiery Consider if patient has an active lifestyle	Consider tolerance and concordance of compression Selection offers below knee and full leg Patient will require aids to apply
Leg assessment	Used to treat leg ulcers Suitable for all sizes of wounds Use with leg ulcers that have moderate to heavy exudate Used for all levels of leg oedema Wadding can be used to reshape leg to achieve correct level of compression at ankle and calf	Use to treat/manage venous leg ulcers Use with low levels of exudate/small ulcers Consider for patients with lower limb oedema Consider in patients with misshapen leg (made-to-measure)	Used to prevent recurrence Made-to-measure may assist with concordance

Wound Care at a Glance, Second Edition. Ian Peate and Melanie Stephens.
© 2020 John Wiley & Sons Ltd. Published 2020 by John Wiley & Sons Ltd.
Companion website: http://www.ataglanceseries.com/nursing/woundcare/

Compression therapy is used to treat venous insufficiency, with or without the presence of venous ulceration. Venous insufficiency is a result of venous hypertension brought about by incompetent non-return valves located on the inside walls of the vein. If treatment is not provided for this condition, the tissue integrity surrounding the affected veins is reduced, and ulceration occurs in some cases.

What is meant by compression?

Compression therapy is the application of a graduated compressive force around the affected limb by using compression bandages (Figure 37.1) or compression hosiery (Figure 37.2). This therapy enhances the functioning of the venous valves, thereby reducing venous hypertension, aiding venous return. This improves the tissue integrity, as waste products and toxins are expressed from the tissues back into the veins for disposal via the correct route (e.g. the kidneys).

There are two types of compression bandage systems: multilayer bandages and short-stretch bandages. The system selected must be applied in accordance with the manufacturer's recommendations, and it should be handled by a health professional trained and competent in the application of this therapy. Compression hosiery is an alternative method of compression; however, it can be difficult to apply to a limb because of the lack of elasticity, thus, it is not the first choice of therapy for a patient with a leg ulcer.

Ultimately, all compression systems are aimed at supporting the structure of vein walls that have become varicosed because of their incompetence. Compression therapy is applied only after a full assessment of the patient is conducted. This includes an examination of the patient's overall health and well-being and a vascular assessment, including a Doppler ultrasound to record the patient's ankle–brachial pressure indices. Patients with a significant degree of arterial insufficiency may suffer harm if compression is applied, reducing the arterial flow. A registered nurse with extended skills ascertains the degree of arterial insufficiency and decides on applying the compression therapy. Therefore, it is essential that the health professional is aware of the contraindications of the compression (refer to table in Chapter 40).

In the UK, the optimum therapeutic level of compression is around 40 mmHg at the ankle, reducing to around 17 mmHg below the knee.

Laplace's Law

The amount of pressure applied to a limb is referred to as Laplace's law; the amount of compression applied can be increased by applying a narrow bandage or by increasing the number of layers applied. If the stress on the bandage (as recommended by the manufacturer) is maintained at the same level, the pressure decreases, as the bandage is wound around the limb, thereby having a huge pressure at the ankle, which then reduces as it rises up to the knee. Box 37.1 shows how the pressures are calculated according to the Laplace's law.

Compression bandaging

Bandages are manufactured as either inelastic (short stretch), elastic (long stretch) or a combination of both materials.

Long stretch bandage systems consist of up to four layers; the top two layers forming the compression layers. By omitting one of the top two layers, there is a reduced level of compression applied. Reduced compression is used in cases where mild peripheral vascular disease may be present, but reduced compression should only be used under specialist supervision. Multilayer systems are suitable for an immobile patient or for those who have an ineffective calf muscle pump, as the pressures remain constant even when immobile. The layers are as follows:

- The first layer consists of absorbent wadding. It protects bone prominences from pressure damage and is used to shape the limb into an inverted 'cone' shape in order to distribute pressure. More padding is used on smaller circumference ankles of less than 18 cm and not greater than 25 cm, in order to achieve up to 40 mmHg pressure around the ankle.
- The second layer is a crepe bandage, which secures the wadding and serves as an additional absorbent layer.
- The third layer consists of an elastic bandage that provides 17 mmHg pressure at the ankle.
- The fourth layer is a cohesive bandage that provides 23 mmHg pressure at the ankle.

Therefore, the third and fourth layers combined provide 40 mmHg compression, and this provides full compression commonly used when there is an ankle–brachial pressure index (ABPI) of >8. The ABPI result determines the requirement of reduced compression (Table 37.1).

When ankle circumference is greater than 25 cm, this reduces the sub-bandage pressure; here, an additional cohesive compression layer will be required, although this would be applied in the opposite direction to the original layer.

Short stretch systems require the patient to be mobile with an effective calf muscle pump, in order to achieve full compression when walking. At rest, the compression will be significantly reduced, so is often more tolerable to patients. These bandages are usually two-layer systems, with wadding being the first layer in order to shape and pad the limb. The second compression layer is applied at full stretch in order to create a firm cylindrical pressure around the limb. When the patient walks, the muscle is forced against the 'cylinder' causing the blood in deeper veins to be compressed, forcing the blood back to the heart.

Compression hosiery

Hosiery is usually used as a maintenance treatment for venous insufficiency to prevent ulcer recurrence and is usually applied once an ulcer is fully healed. Standard sizes and made-to-measure are available with different classes of compression that apply different levels of compression at the ankle (Table 37.1). Patients wearing hosiery or bandages must only do so under medical advice, and they must have their ABPI monitored on a regular basis (e.g. trimonthly). Some manufactures have developed two-layer hosiery kits for ease of application due to the inner layer providing a smoother surface than the skin.

Person-centred therapy

It is well documented that patients find compression therapy very difficult to concord with. This is because bandages are bulky; stockings are difficult to apply; the therapy makes the patient hot; and, initially, there is an increase in pain levels when applied to an oedematous limb with an ulcer. The psychological impact of an ulcer and the additional problems of pain, such as wet and leaking bandages and malodour, are some other issues.

To reduce the possibility of non-concordance, it is recommended that the affected limb be measured accurately to safeguard a good fit, and aids should be recommended to assist with the application of hosiery. The right compression therapy should reduce oedema and pain, as the ulcer begins to heal; however, it is good practice to review any analgesia taken by the patient.

Healing of an ulcer does not occur with compression therapy alone. Therefore, it is important to educate the patient about venous disease; the role of compression therapy in treatment; and prevention and health advice in regard to leg elevation, foot exercises, nutrition, sleep, hygiene and pain management.

38 Arterial ulcers

Figure 38.1 Arterial ulcer.

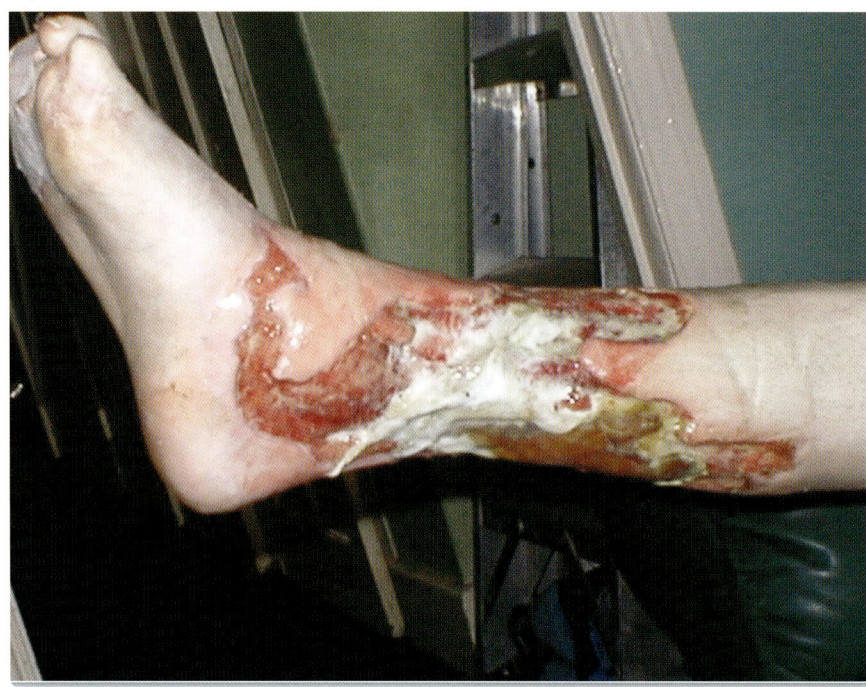

Figure 38.2 Arteriosclerosis.

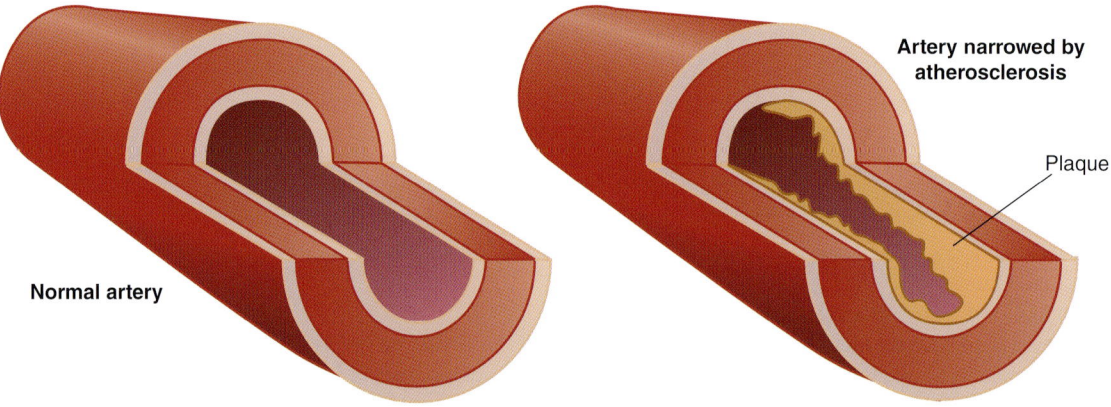

Source: P. Vong. Reproduced with permission of P. Vong.

Arterial insufficiency

Arterial insufficiency, often called 'peripheral arterial disease' (PAD), is the lack of, or a reduction in, the blood supply. It is found in varying degrees of severity among sufferers, ranging from mild PAD to critical ischaemia (i.e. tissue death due to no blood supply). PAD of the lower extremities accounts for around 10% of all leg ulceration in the UK. However, a leg ulcer could be of venous, arterial or mixed (i.e. both arterial and venous) aetiology, and it is important to identify the type of ulcer being treated, as the treatments required for different types of ulcers are very different. It is vital that priority consideration be given to the presence of PAD while considering treatment. The causes, diagnosis and treatment of venous ulcers are explained in previous chapters. In this chapter, we will look at the causes, diagnosis and treatments of arterial ulceration (Figure 38.1).

Aetiology and risk factors

Blood circulates from the heart to every cell in the body via the arterial system; first via larger arteries (e.g. aorta), then branching into smaller main arteries, then into smaller arteries and then into capillaries, which are found at the tip of the arterial tree. Arterial blood delivers oxygen and nutrients to cells to maintain health and life, without which tissues die.

There are many reasons why arterial insufficiency occurs, including arteriosclerosis (plaque development in the lumen of the artery/capillary, Figure 38.2); destruction of capillaries from disease (e.g. diabetes), from smoking and from high blood pressure (hypertension); trauma, and/or unrelieved pressure; and from age-related changes that cause vasoconsolidation (hardening of the arteries) or vasoconstriction (narrowing).

Medical conditions – for example, coronary heart disease, diabetes, stroke and vascular diseases (such as vascular dementia or organ failure due to vascular disease) – make it more probable for the patient to also develop PAD. Additionally, any patient with PAD is at an increased risk of developing pressure ulcers (discussed earlier).

In PAD, it is common for the tip of the arterial tree to be affected first, so the skin and the extremities, and their underlying tissues, will be at risk of tissue death. This can result in reduced tissue integrity in the mildest of cases, to onset of or the non-healing of existing wounds. In the severest conditions, it can result in gangrene of the limb (e.g. commonly in the toes/feet in diabetics) due to the complete occlusion of one or more arteries. The tissues that will be affected will depend on which artery (or arteries) or capillaries are blocked.

Symptoms

It is most common for symptoms to have an insidious onset to begin with, whereby no symptoms are obvious. However, there are occasions when a sudden blockage of an artery will occur that causes excruciating ischaemic pain for the individual. For patients with the former type of PAD, the symptoms gradually increase over time and can include one or more of the following classic signs:

- Thin, shiny, hairless legs (or patches of hair loss).
- Thickened toenails (reduced blood supply to the nail bed).
- Pale, cool feet (pales and cools further on limb elevation).
- Foot discolouration (can be very red, or black).
- Poor tissue perfusion (i.e. capillary refill >4 seconds). Capillary refill time reduces on limb elevation.
- Weak or absent foot pulses (sounds heard on Doppler may fade on limb elevation).
- Limb pain that worsens on limb elevation and is relieved by lowering the limb.
- Pain on walking, relieved by resting (intermittent claudication).
- Severe pain on resting.
- Non-healing leg wounds that have a deep, punched-out appearance with steep edges.

Diagnosis

As always, diagnosis is made following holistic and clinical assessment of the limb. A Doppler ABPI (ankle–brachial pressure index) assessment can be carried out to confirm the nurse's suspicions of vascular disease; however, this may not be tolerated well by the patient due to the pain likely to be experienced. In cases where an ABPI is obtained that is outside of the normal range of 1.0–1.2, the patient should be referred to a vascular team for further assessment and a duplex scan should be done in order to determine the extent of the PAD and the most appropriate treatment. Where a normal range ABPI is obtained, but the patient experiences any of the above symptoms, PAD must be considered as a possibility. In the meantime, where PAD is suspected based on assessment findings, care must be taken to avoid any compression therapy, tight clothing or footwear until the patient is assessed by the vascular team.

Treatment

Treatment options vary depending on the findings and severity of the PAD. In many cases, an angioplasty can be performed to stretch/sweep the narrowed artery to increase blood flow. This often produces temporary improvements, and repeat angioplasties are necessary. Occasionally, where larger arteries are blocked or narrowed, surgery can be performed in order to remove the blockage or to reroute the arteries by way of bypass grafts. However, in cases where it is the capillaries that are blocked or damaged, no treatment is available, and it is a case of treating the patient holistically by providing education on lifestyle choices and skin care. This may include exercise therapy, where patients are encouraged to learn how to walk through the pain to stimulate the growth of new blood vessels. Patients are supported to walk for 30 minutes three times a week, exercising at least to the point of maximum pain and up to 2 hours supervised walking per week.

It is essential that best practice in wound care be provided, so that the wound can heal as quickly as possible, at rates that are determined by the level of blood supply to the wound bed. In many cases, a wound fails to heal regardless of the applied treatments because there is insufficient blood supply to the wound bed. This may include recent advances in the use of compression therapy; however, this treatment plan is undertaken by an expert practitioner who is aware of the benefits and risks of the application of compression on a patient with peripheral arterial disease.

39 Assessing for arterial disease: ankle–brachial pressure index and toe–brachial pressure index

Figure 39.1 Non-bleeding visible vessel.

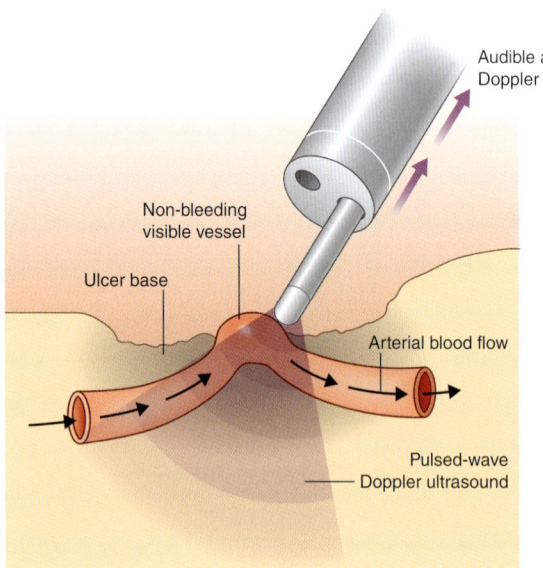

Figure 39.3 Some Dopplers also produce a visual wave form reading.

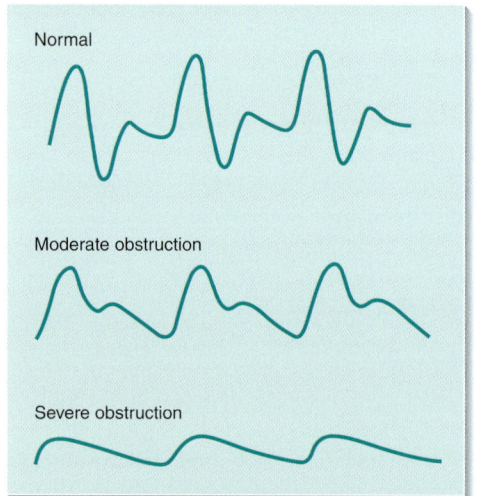

Figure 39.2 Doppler equipment and application.

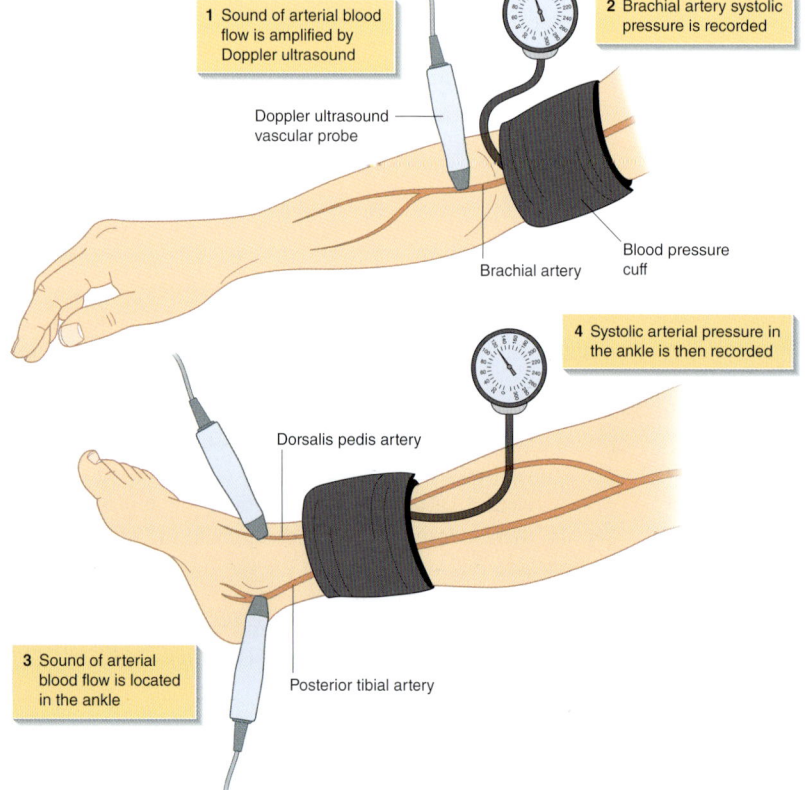

Box 39.1 Doppler ultrasound signals.

Triphasic signal
Represented by three sounds heard very quickly together (duh…duh…duh); occurs as the blood rushes through a healthy artery.

Biphasic signal
Two sounds heard together (duh…duh), indicating a healthy artery; the Doppler probe may not be at the optimum angle.

Monophasic signal
This is almost a single banging sound, indicating that the Doppler signal cannot penetrate a diseased artery. This sound is usually lower in pitch.

Box 39.2 TBPI results.

TBPI score	Result implication
TBPI >0.7	Normal peripheral arterial supply.
TBPI <0.65	Suggestive of peripheral arterial disease. Refer patient to the vascular team.

Wound Care at a Glance, Second Edition. Ian Peate and Melanie Stephens.
© 2020 John Wiley & Sons Ltd. Published 2020 by John Wiley & Sons Ltd.
Companion website: http://www.ataglanceseries.com/nursing/woundcare/

As 1% of the population is affected by leg ulceration and 5–7% of diabetics have a foot ulcer, it is imperative to make a reliable diagnosis in case of a full leg ulcer or foot assessment. This requires the nurse to have knowledge and understanding of the circulatory system of the lower limb and foot, how leg and foot ulcers occur and what monitors or devices can be used to ensure that the right treatment pathway is followed. Common medical devices used in the assessment of leg ulcers or wounds of the lower limb and foot include: ankle–brachial pressure index (ABPI), toe–brachial pressure index, pulse oximetry, two-point tests and plethysmography.

ABPI

A method of undertaking an ABPI is through the use of a hand-held Doppler ultrasound. It is a non-invasive test that measures the blood flow through the blood vessels of the lower leg by bouncing high-frequency sound waves (ultrasound) off circulating red blood cells. Community nurses, for example, calculate the ABPI of a patient by measuring the systolic blood pressure to both arms (brachial) and the ankle at two pulse sites and carrying out a calculation. Generally, all stages of peripheral arterial disease should be verified and confirmed using objective tests, such as the ABPI. Laser Doppler technology is a non-invasive method and is an investigative tool. A laser light is used to detect blood perfusion in the microcirculation (Figure 39.1). The measuring depth is approximately 0.5–1 mm, reaching the superficial vessels:

- Arterioles
- Venules
- Shunts
- Capillaries.

Doppler relates to the change in frequency of a wave, as the source or target moves. When used as part of a vascular assessment, the technique uses the direction and velocity of blood flow to determine whether the patient's arterial blood vessels are healthy or diseased. The brachial and ankle systolic pressures are measured using a hand-held Doppler probe at the brachial pulse and the dorsalis pedis pulse on the dorsum of the foot. The ankle pressure is divided by the brachial pressure to obtain the ABPI.

Performing doppler

The practitioner must provide information that the patients can understand and that is relevant to their circumstances, enabling them to make an informed decision. The information should include details of the possible benefits and risks. Treatment should take into account factors such as physical or learning disabilities, sight or hearing problems, and/or difficulties with reading or speaking English, and appropriate adjustments made.

Patient preparation

The patient should be asked to lie as flat as possible, with one pillow for the head, and the procedure should take 10–20 minutes, assuming this position removes the effect of gravity on blood flow. If the patient is unable to undertake this position, he/she should be asked to lie as low as possible and the legs should be at the level of the heart. This position should be documented in the notes, so that when the Doppler is repeated in future staff can replicate the same position and provide consistency in future recordings. The patient may experience some discomfort, as the blood pressure cuff is placed on the ankle and it is inflated. If at any time the patient finds the procedure too painful, he/she can ask for it to stop at any time. The patient should remove any tight items of clothing, which may cause pressure on the blood vessels proximal to the site where the blood pressure is being measured. The practitioner must remove any dressings from the ulcer and cover it with vapour-permeable film dressing or equivalent to reduce risk of cross-infection.

Equipment required

The following equipment is required (see Figure 39.2):

- A Doppler ultrasound with an 8 Mhz or 5 Mhz probe, if the lower limb is oedematous.
- A sphygmomanometer and the appropriate size blood pressure cuff for the shape and size of the patient's arms and ankles. When the cuff is too short or narrow, the pressures might be overestimated, whereas a cuff that is too big underestimates the pressures.
- Sterile cover to the ulcer bed (helps in preventing the cuff from irritating the ulcer bed, promoting comfort and preventing contamination of the cuff), vapour-permeable film dressing or equivalent.
- Ultrasound gel, used as a contact medium between the patient and the Doppler probe.
- Chart for recording pressures.

The procedure

Two practitioners should work together to perform the procedure, one of whom should be trained in Doppler use and assessment. The patient should be asked to lie flat for 10–20 minutes prior to beginning the procedure (unless contraindicated); this helps to avoid the unwanted effect of gravity.

Apply the blood pressure cuff to the upper arm. The brachial artery should be located through palpation, and transducer gel should be applied to that area. The Doppler probe should be held at 45° pointing towards the heart, over the area of skin that has the gel on it, and the probe should be moved until the clearest signal is located. A continuous whooshing sound means that the vessel is not an artery. It is important to become familiar with sounds of arteries; Box 39.1 explains the different sounds arteries can make depending on the degree of peripheral arterial disease. The blood pressure cuff should be inflated until the signal disappears, and then the cuff should be slowly deflated to listen to the signal to re-emerge; this must be recorded. The same test must be carried out on the other arm, and the highest pressure should be recorded as the brachial systolic pressure, which is compared against the ankle pressures.

The ulcer should be exposed and covered in a vapour-permeable film dressing or equivalent. The pedal arteries should be located. There are four of these:

1. Anterior tibial artery
2. Posterior tibial artery
3. Peroneal artery
4. Dorsalis pedis artery.

Two of the four are used; the most common ones are the most accessible: the dorsalis pedis and the posterior tibial arteries. The blood pressure cuff is tied above the malleoli; the transducer gel is applied over the artery. The Doppler is applied over the artery, and the best signal is detected. The blood pressure cuff is slowly inflated. The disappearing Doppler signal should be listened to, as the pressure exerted in the cuff occludes the artery. The cuff should be slowly deflated; the pressure at which the Doppler signal reappears must be observed and noted; this pressure for that artery should be recorded. The patient should be enquired on now. One of the other pedal arteries should be located, and the process should be repeated. If the blood pressure cuff cannot compress the artery, this is an indication of severe disease (see Figure 39.3 and Box 39.1).

After obtaining all of the readings, the patient must be made comfortable while slowly assisting him/her to take the upright position. The patient must be informed of what has been done and what will happen next. The practitioner must perform Doppler ultrasound in addition to obtaining a detailed health history, and this should incorporate the patient's social circumstances.

All findings should be recorded.

Automated ABPI

Automated devices have been manufactured that simplify and quicken the recording of the ABPI in comparison to hand-held devices. The recording and measuring of the ABPI using the automated device mean that resting is no longer required; only one person is required to carry out the assessment, and the three-cuff method increases the accuracy of results. Initial training and education are required, and a limitation is that staff can become deskilled from using hand-held devices. All findings should be recorded.

Toe–brachial pressure index (TBPI)

In some instances, the practitioner may be required to undertake a Doppler ultrasound to measure toe pressures. This may be when the ABPI records false high readings, owing to calcification of the arteries, there is gross oedema of the leg, or the patient experiences pain and discomfort when carrying out an ABPI. As calcification seldom affects the toe arteries, TBPI may be carried out. Most TBPIs are conducted using a Vascular Assist machine® or with an appropriately sized cuff and a hand-held Doppler. The measurement is toe pressure divided by the highest brachial pressure (see Box 39.2).

Pressures in the toe are lesser than those in the ankle, and the readings are interpreted differently. The recordings should be documented.

Pulse oximetry

Pulse oximeters measure oxygen levels within the tissue, and the signal is diminished when blood flow is occluded. The pulse oximeter is placed on the finger or toe, and the cuff is placed around the arm or ankle, depending on which reading is being taken. Training is required in the application and inflation of the blood pressure cuff. The calculation is the same as ABPI and TBPI, toe level divided by highest finger reading.

Compression ultrasound

Compression ultrasound venous imaging is a non-invasive test for the diagnosis of deep vein thrombosis (DVT). In a two-point test, the ability of the ultrasound probe to compress the common femoral vein and popliteal vein is assessed by using two-dimensional ultrasound image display. Normal veins are compressible, whereas those containing thrombi are not. If both are compressible, the examination is considered negative. In a three-point examination, the femoral vein is also examined, as it increases diagnostic sensitivity and accuracy of a DVT.

Plethysmography

Limb plethysmography is a test that compares blood pressure in the legs and arms. The patient is asked to lie down with the upper body slightly raised. Three or four blood pressure cuffs are applied to the patient's arm and leg (depending on the device type). The practitioner inflates the cuffs, and a machine called a 'plethysmograph' measures the pulses from each cuff. The test records the maximum pressure produced when the heart contracts (systolic blood pressure). Differences between the pulses are noted. If there is a decrease in the pulse between the arm and leg, it may indicate a blockage.

Heel pressure ulcers

Peripheral arterial disease (PAD) is a common risk factor for the development of heel pressure ulcers. However, PAD may neither be recorded in the patient's notes nor diagnosed. Simple diagnostic assessments that can aid risk assessment include: assessing capillary refill time, palpation of pulses in the foot, ankle–brachial pressure index and peripheral sensory screening tests. These tests are usually carried out by a trained practitioner, and decisions can be made on using preventative aids to redistribute pressure or off-load the heels, such as pressure-redistributing mattresses, heel lift devices and heel protectors. Patients who have pressure ulcers and whose ABPI measures a degree of PAD require a referral to the vascular surgeon.

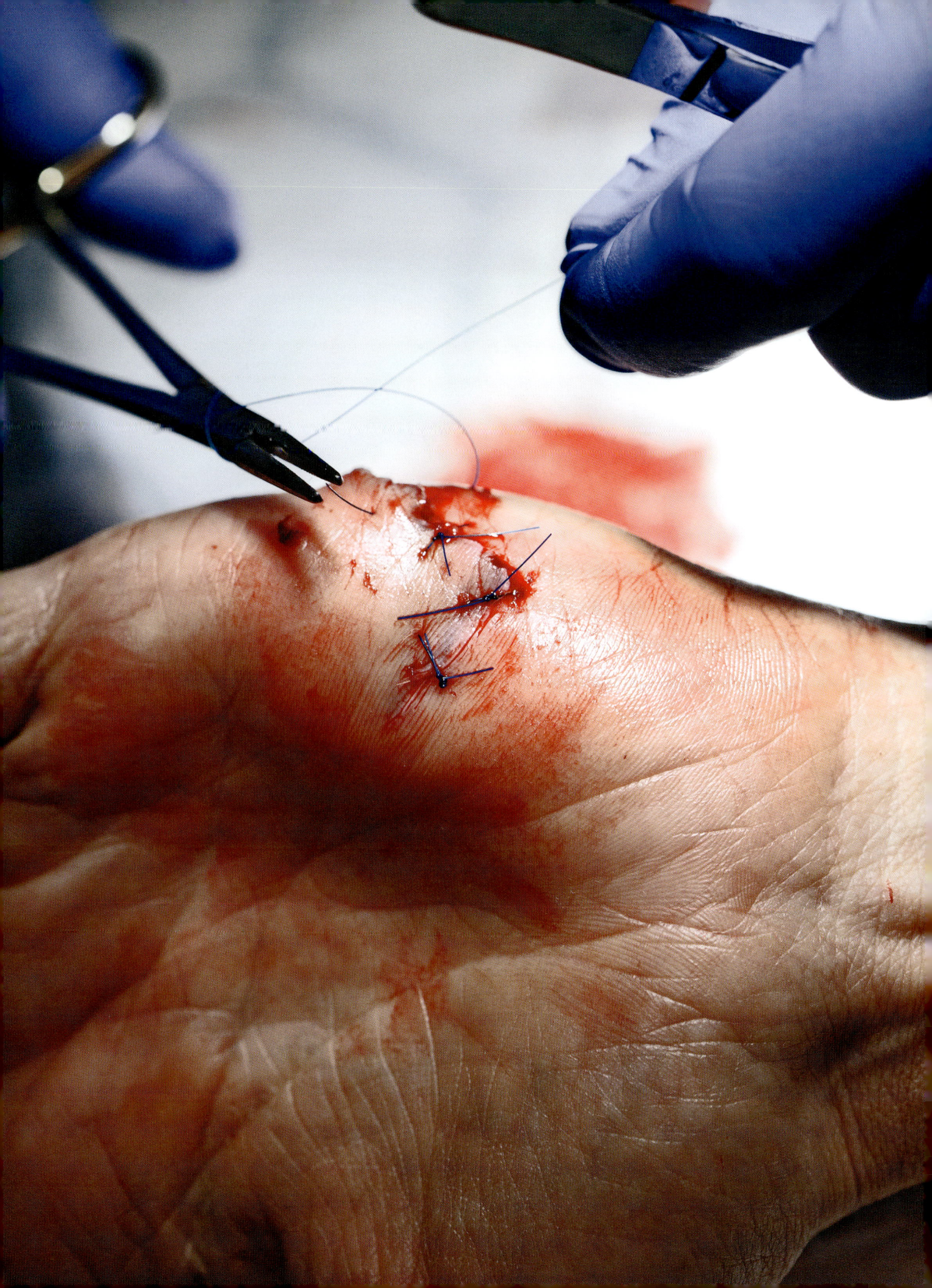

40 Interpreting ABPIs

Table 40.1 ABPI and clinical indicators for compression therapy.

ABPI	Clinical indication	Therapy advised
1.0–1.3	No indicators of PAD	Apply high level of compression
0.8–1.0	Mild PAD	May use high compression, but regularly monitor ABPI
0.51–0.8	Significant PAD	May use reduced compression – refer to leg ulcer/vascular nurse specialist
<0.5	Severe PAD	No compression – urgent referral to vascular surgeon
>1.3	Measure toe pressures/refer to specialist	May use compression – refer to leg ulcer/vascular nurse specialist

Wound Care at a Glance, Second Edition. Ian Peate and Melanie Stephens.
© 2020 John Wiley & Sons Ltd. Published 2020 by John Wiley & Sons Ltd.
Companion website: http://www.ataglanceseries.com/nursing/woundcare/

An ABPI result must not be considered in isolation when it comes to the management of leg ulcers; however, it does confirm or rule out any vascular disease, which indicates when not to apply compression therapy. When performing a Doppler assessment, it is equally, if not more, important to undertake a full examination of the entire limb for signs of underlying conditions that may indicate vascular or venous disease. It is also important to ask the patient about pain and any aggravating factors that may exacerbate pain. By conducting a full assessment, the nurse can ascertain the cause of the ulcer, factors that impact on wound healing and aetiology of the ulcer.

Table 40.1 considers ABPI results and clinical indications to guide the nurse on the most appropriate management for the patient.

A Doppler and recording of a patient's ankle–brachial pressure indices is one part of the process and aids assessment of arterial disease in the lower leg. The procedure must, however, be conducted correctly to reduce potential incorrect diagnosis and harmful/ineffective treatment.

The foot pulses must be located and the sounds of the blood flow must be listened to, as this can determine how healthy the arteries actually are and whether or not the ulcer is likely to be of arterial or venous origin. Secondly, the ABPI result determines whether or not compression therapy is appropriate, or whether a referral to a vascular surgeon is appropriate on an urgent basis or not.

Artery sounds

1. *Triphasic sounds*: These are audible by Doppler ultrasound, as the vessel expands and relaxes in rhythm with the heart beat and blood circulation. A triphasic beat indicates a healthy artery.
2. *Biphasic sound*: As blood reaches the lower extremities (i.e. the feet), the sound fades; in older adults, only two beats may be heard. A biphasic beat can indicate that the arteries are beginning to harden but can be considered as a normal physiological process of aging.
3. *Monophasic sound*: If only one beat is heard (usually a loud whooshing sound), this indicates a calcified (hardened) vessel. The walls are less elastic than a healthy artery, often due to age or disease, such as diabetes. The sound is often much louder than a healthy artery, as the blood flow causes echoing within the artery.

Monophasic-sounding arteries

The monophasic beat is an indication that the blood vessel is unhealthy, and the causes of this can be:

- Stenosis of the artery from the consequences of atherosclerosis causing peripheral vascular disease.
- Arteriovenous fistula (an abnormal connection between an artery and a vein in the leg).
- Arteriovenous malformation (an abnormal connection between arteries and veins, bypassing capillaries).
- Inflammatory processes that create oedema in the lower limb.
- Exercise.

When a vessel is compressed, the cut-off and re-entry sound pressures must be noted; the sound of a healthy artery will cut off and re-enter at the same mmHg pressure, whereas a stenosed or calcified vessel will have a different sound of re-entry than the point at which the vessel was completely occluded. This is because a healthy artery is more flexible and occludes easier with direct pressure than a calcified artery, which is harder to occlude and slower to spring open, thereby causing the delay in sound re-entry.

Monophasic sounds can be lower in pitch than biphasic and triphasic sounds (stenosis) and can be described like soldiers marching (rigid vessels) or a howling sound.

ABPI results and referral pathway

All ABPI results must be interpreted by registered health professionals within the context of their roles and responsibilities, education and training, local policy, the patient's full health, well-being, leg ulcer assessment and Doppler results.

A normal ABPI is regarded as being above 1, provided there are no other clinical signs of any vascular disease; compression therapy is usually recommended.

For ABPI above 1.3, or if compression above 180 mmHg pressure is required to occlude, the artery sound is usually indicative of calcified vessels. Compression ought to be avoided until the patient is assessed by a leg ulcer specialist.

An ABPI between 0.8 and 1 denotes mild peripheral artery disease (PAD), but does not usually require any intervention, provided there are no other clinical signs of arterial compromise. It is usually acceptable to apply compression therapy; however, close monitoring of the ABPI and clinical inspection of the limb must be undertaken on a regular basis (e.g. monthly) to observe for deterioration in the vascular status of the limb.

ABPIs between 0.5 and 0.8 indicate that there is a moderate peripheral arterial disease of the lower limb. The urgency of the referral depends on the result. There may be associated pain on limb elevation or on walking (claudication). A leg ulcer specialist or a vascular nurse may decide to manage the patient's lower limb/ulcers with compression therapy. This requires close monitoring.

When the ABPI is <0.5 and/or if foot pulses are absent, it will be common for the patient to complain of severe resting pain, which collectively may be indicative of critical ischaemia and may require an urgent referral for further investigation and opinion.

Calculating ABPIs

When calculating ABPIs, it is common practice that the highest brachial pulse is used to calculate the ABPI against all pulses. Similarly, it is the highest foot pulse that is used to calculate the ABPI on each foot. However, care must be taken not to overlook the lowest foot pulse on each foot, as this could indicate that that particular vessel is partially occluded, and using the highest foot pulse could mask a problem in the neighbouring artery.

A nurse who undertakes an ABPI should be well-trained and competent, since an incorrect calculation or procedure could lead to inappropriate or contraindicated care being provided. Incorrect treatment could lead to increased pain, delayed healing or compromised circulation in the event that compression therapy is applied when it ought to be contraindicated.

41 Diabetic foot ulcers

Figure 41.1 Diabetic leg and foot ulcers.

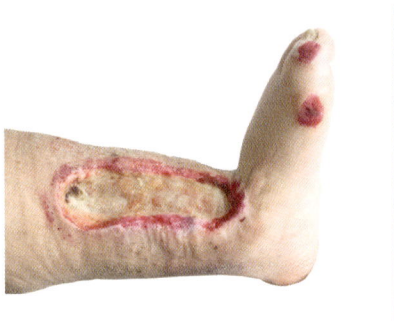

Source: Shutterstock © Svitlana Kazachek.

Figure 41.2 Pressure ulcer on the diabetic foot.

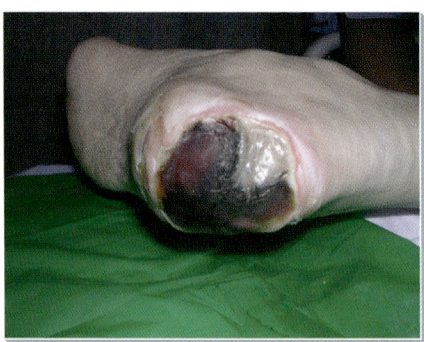

Figure 41.3 Sloughy neuropathic foot ulcer.

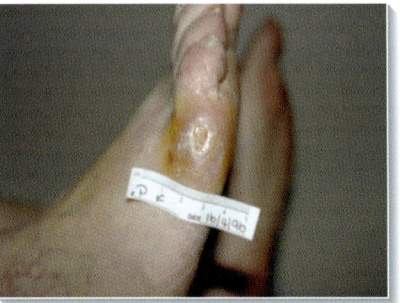

Figure 41.4 Neuropathic foot ulcer after maggot therapy.

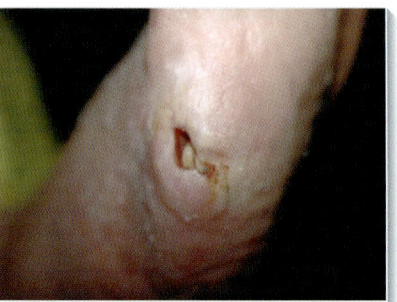

Figure 41.5 Diabetic foot ulcers with gangrenous (black) areas.

(a)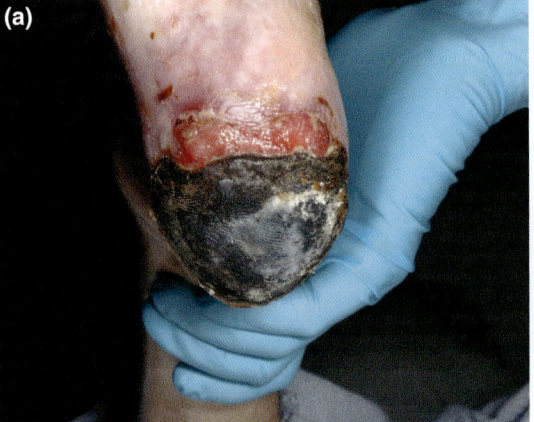

(b)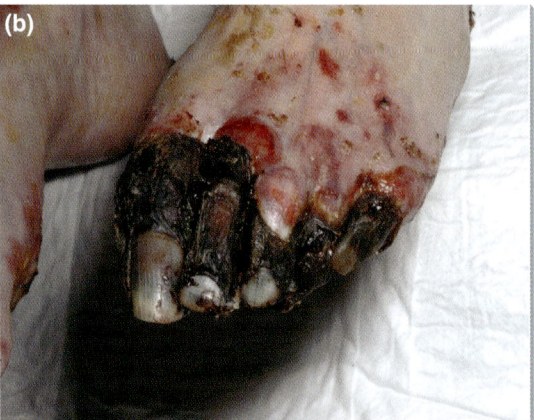

Wound Care at a Glance, Second Edition. Ian Peate and Melanie Stephens.
© 2020 John Wiley & Sons Ltd. Published 2020 by John Wiley & Sons Ltd.
Companion website: http://www.ataglanceseries.com/nursing/woundcare/

Diabetes is a condition where the pancreas either fails to produce sufficient insulin, or not at all, and sugar levels in the blood increase as a result. This in turn causes destruction of blood vessels, from activities such as reduced levels of nitric oxide (a powerful vasodilator), thereby causing narrowing of the arteries and many conditions as a consequence. For example, patients with diabetes have an increased risk of conditions such as dementia, vascular disease, multiorgan failure, glaucoma and loss of sight – and, in terms of tissue viability, foot and leg ulcers (Figure 41.1) that could potentially lead to amputation.

Diabetes has two types (Type I and Type II); the risk of the latter increases with age and obesity, and it is becoming an increasing phenomenon in the developed world, with more people developing Type II diabetes than ever before.

The diabetic patient can develop a foot ulcer (DFU) spontaneously; also, in the event that a wound occurs for other reasons (e.g. surgery, trauma and pressure), they are notoriously difficult to heal. Furthermore, the risk of infection is increased in a diabetic person due to the reduction in blood supply (and therefore white blood cells) to the wound bed. Currently, 5–7% of all diabetic patients have a foot ulcer, and almost 25% develop a foot ulcer in their lifetime. A DFU is a critical event in the life of a diabetic patient, signifying serious health issues and overall well-being. Early interprofessional intervention is key to the prevention and management of this potentially life-changing and/or life-threatening illness. Peripheral neuropathy and peripheral arterial disease play a dominant role, and DFUs are classified as neuropathic, ischaemic or neuroischaemic.

The diabetic patient often develops neuropathy, affecting sensory, motor and autonomic nerves. This means that the patient does not feel the pain of any physical, chemical or thermal trauma. The neuropathy may lead to the development of foot deformities, such as hammer and claw toes, or dry skin with cracks, fissures and callus.

A diabetic patient is also twice prone to develop a peripheral arterial disease than a non-diabetic patient. Poor perfusion of the lower limb can lead to delayed wound healing.

This often means that diabetic foot wounds are overlooked until such time that they become saturated with exudate and/or become infected, and a malodour is noted by the patient. Prevention is therefore much better than cure.

Foot surveillance, foot checks and foot care

First and foremost, it is crucial that a diabetic patient undergoes regular (annual) foot checks with a diabetic podiatrist so that the structure, sensation and vascular status can be monitored in accordance with best practice. The patient or care staff should thereafter monitor the patient's feet for signs of callus (hard skin) that may have underlying ulcers, for any signs of trauma (e.g. from footwear) and for the onset of any wounds that may occur spontaneously. In any such event, it is crucial to provide excellence in wound management and to ensure that a prompt referral to a diabetic foot specialist is made without any delay. A patient should be seen within one working day of the presentation of the ulcer, preferably by a multidisciplinary diabetic foot team (MDFT), or sooner in case of severe infection.

It is crucial that correct-fitting footwear be used, and the diabetic podiatrist/MDFT will be best placed to give advice on this.

Foot complications

Diabetic patients have an increased risk of developing pressure ulcers due to their compromised circulation and the possible presence of neuropathy, which means they are unable to respond to the effects of pressure, so will remain in the same position, thereby compromising the circulation further, causing necrosis (tissue death), as can be seen in Figures 41.2–41.4.

As a diabetic patient's foot structure changes, he/she can develop a condition called *Charcot osteoarthropathy*, which causes the instep to collapse as the bone structures collapse, often causing the appearance of flat feet or a 'rocker' sole, which then makes the patient more vulnerable to pressure damage; thus, observation of the foot and prompt referral is vital to prevent wounds occurring.

Wound assessment

Patients with a DFU require a full assessment, which includes patient history, medication, comorbidities and diabetes status. It should also include the history of the wound, previous DFUs or amputations and any symptoms of neuropathy or PAD. The podiatrist assesses the ulcer, performs a wound assessment, tests for loss of sensation, checks vascular status, identifies any infection, inspects the feet for deformities and classifies the DFU. By completing a holistic assessment, a clear wound management plan can be prescribed.

Wound management

Essential to wound management of the DFU are: treatment of the underlying disease processes; ensuring adequate blood supply; wound care of the ulcer and peri-wound area; infection control; and the offloading of pressure. This may include one off or frequent debridement of the wound (performed by an experienced practitioner – e.g. specialist podiatrist, nurse or vascular surgeon with specialist training), control of bacteria at the wound bed and management of exudate to prevent maceration and excoriation. The TIME framework is useful for managing DFUs.

Due to the increased risk of wound infection and, often, the presence of tissue death (gangrene), there are some very important points that require discussion:

- *Gangrene*: This is caused by dead tissues due to lack of blood supply and is often a feature of a diabetic foot ulcer (Figure 41.5). The lack of oxygen causes ischaemia and subsequent tissue death. The gangrene can appear as dry gangrene (black, necrotic appearance) or wet gangrene (green, sloughy appearance). The tissues continue to die until they get a healthy blood supply, after which the gangrene usually autoamputates, provided it is allowed to remain dry (or is dried out), and the wound then heals at that point. It can affect one part of the foot (e.g. one toe), or the entire foot (also involving the leg), and may, in critical cases, require surgical amputation in the event of increased pain or the risk of gas gangrene.
- *Gas gangrene*: This is a dead tissue that is affected by a gas-producing bacterium known as *Clostridium perfringens*. The gas produced by the bacterium liquefies and then breaks down the tissues, which can then rapidly place the patient's limb or life at risk. This particular bacterium thrives in moist to wet environments and is unable to survive in dry environments. Indeed, this bacterium is present in most soils on earth except in deserts, and it is responsible for decomposing dead bodies. Bodies have been preserved in desert sands for thousands of years because this bacterium does not exist in deserts. Therefore, where gangrene exists in an ischaemic limb (including any other necrotic tissues), care must be taken to dry out the affected tissues in order to prevent the rapid production of this bacteria, and the potential to destroy a limb or cause the patient's death by sepsis is often within 24–48 hours.
- *The treatment of gangrene is dependent on whether it is dry, wet or gas gangrene, and can include*: surgery to repair and bypass

damaged blood vessels; antibiotics and antimicrobial dressings to treat the infection; debridement of the wound using either sharp debridement, larvae therapy or autolytic debridement using dressings; and hyperbaric oxygen therapy.

- *Moist wound healing*: This is contraindicated in the gangrenous wound; it is only recommended when there is a wound bed that is free from gangrene (or any other necrotic tissue – e.g. black slough/debris) and when the blood supply to the wound bed is very good. If the blood supply is good to the wound bed, the immunity will be good (via the white blood cells), providing the diabetic patient some protection from infection. General principles in wound management apply in the DFU; however, many dressings used in other types of wound may not be suitable. As the status of a DFU can rapidly change (e.g. if an infection is not appropriately assessed), regular inspection and assessment of the ulcer are required. Therefore, dressings that can be left in place for more than 5 days are not usually appropriate for a DFU. Most DFU dressings are changed once daily to once in 2–3 days, dependent on assessment of tissues at the wound bed, infection and levels of exudate. A multi-disciplinary foot team working with a podiatrist advising on treatment is essential, with inspection at regular intervals.

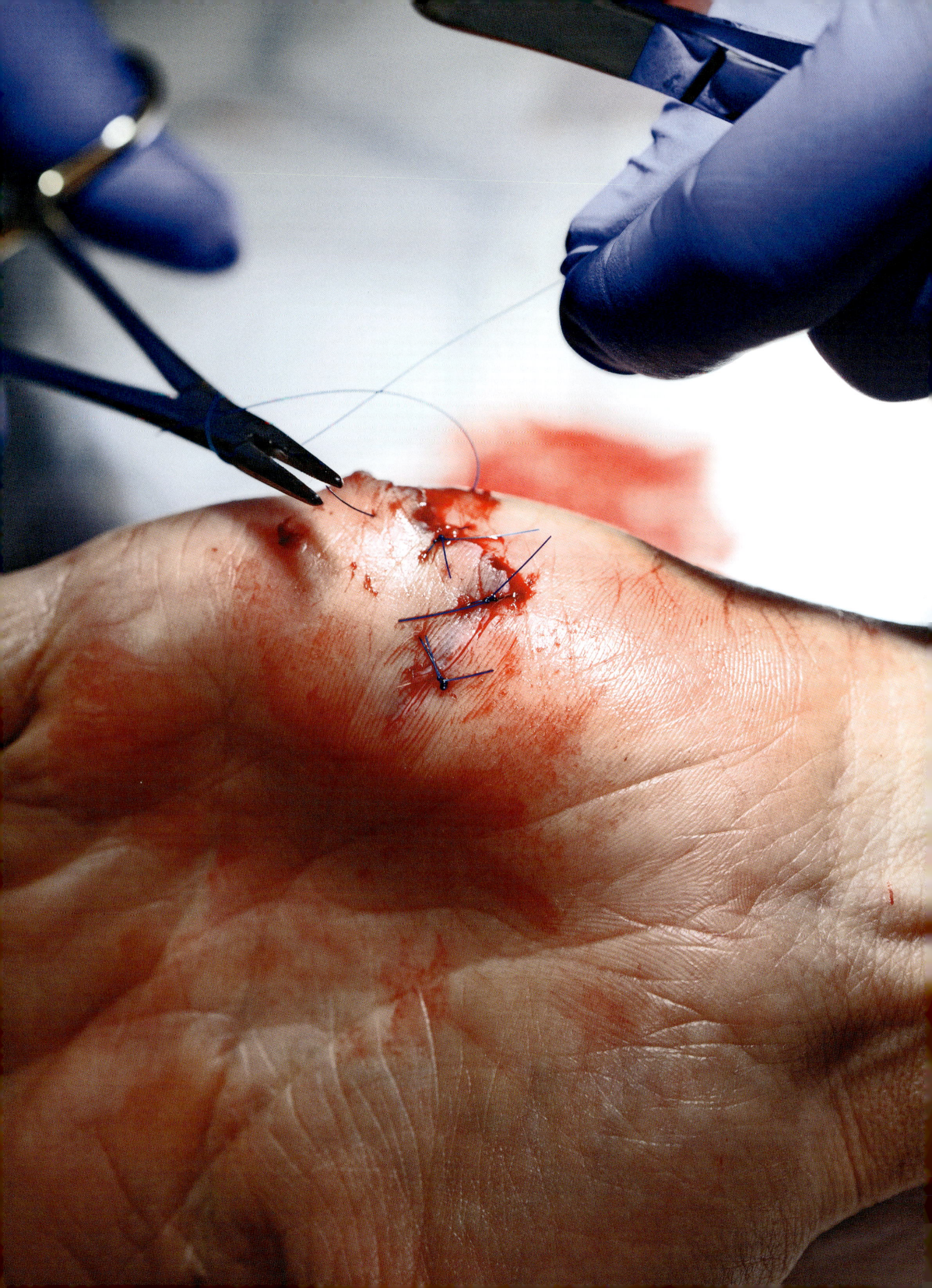

42 Moisture lesions

Figure 42.1 Moisture lesion on the buttocks.

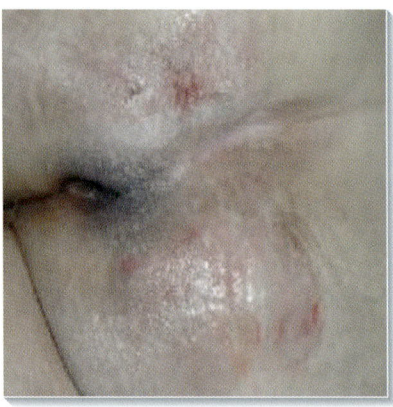

Figure 42.2 Blanching erythema.

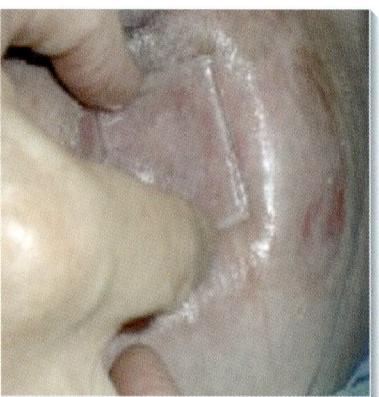

Figure 42.3 Non-blanching erythema. Grades 1, 2 and 3 pressure damage.

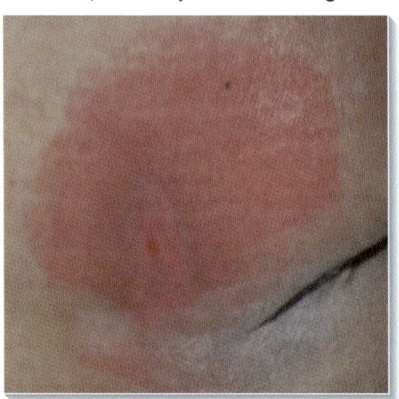

Figure 42.4 Grade 4 pressure damage.

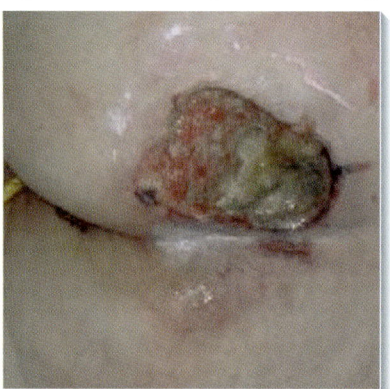

Table 42.1 Differences between moisture lesions and pressure ulcers.

Pressure ulcer	Moisture lesion
Usually occurs over a bony prominence, such as over the sacrum, or under anything that applies constant pressure to the skin, for example, under the tight elastic on underwear, or medical device	Occurs where there is excess moisture against the skin. The area may be extensive, and over areas where there are no bones immediately underneath the skin, for example, the buttocks, groin and folds of skin on the thighs, abdomen, under the breasts, etc. The skin initially looks wet and shiny.
Distinct edges or margins usually round in shape to begin with, and are confined to the area directly over the bone	Appears initially as a rash or a tiny graze(s) that are sporadic over the area of moisture. Poorly defined edges may be blotchy.
The onset of pressure damage appears red (when it is Category 1). When pressed, it is non-blanching (i.e. it remains red when pressed, Figure 42.3)	Appears red, and the red area blanches when pressed (i.e. it goes white)
The skin surrounding the ulcer is usually dry	The skin around the lesions appears 'wet'
The depth of damage can go deep down to the muscle, bones and tendons	Is usually superficial, although if combined with pressure, the damage can go deep as with pressure ulcers. These ulcers are categorised as combined ulcers. Kissing ulcers and a linear wound to the anal cleft can develop.
Can become infected, although this is unusual with good wound management. Therefore, any infection gets delayed, if at all	Can usually become infected very quickly due to the presence of bodily fluids and matter that harbours bacterial growth
Usually hot or lumpy to touch	Usually cool to touch, unless infected
The patient complains of pain	The patient usually complains of a stinging sensation, tingling, burning and itching

Wound Care at a Glance, Second Edition. Ian Peate and Melanie Stephens.
© 2020 John Wiley & Sons Ltd. Published 2020 by John Wiley & Sons Ltd.
Companion website: http://www.ataglanceseries.com/nursing/woundcare/

Moisture lesions are the areas of the skin that are damaged by excessive and prolonged contact with moisture, such as sweat, incontinence of faeces and urine, from wound exudate or from spillages (Figure 42.1). Initially the skin becomes wet, and the dead skin cells absorb the moisture. This then causes the skin to become macerated (i.e. soggy or water-logged). Eventually, the maceration reaches the cuboidal cells rendering them penetrable by bacteria, and so the skin is breached and an open wound occurs. The resulting skin damage is usually very superficial and usually destroys the epidermal and the dermal layers of the skin (Figures 42.2 and 42.3). The severity of the damage depends on the extent that the moisture spreads, and so can often result in widespread destruction (Figure 42.4). This type of wound occurs commonly under skinfolds, such as under the breasts, under the abdominal apron, around the buttocks, groin, sacrum and vulval areas. As a result, fungal infections commonly occur on these lesions, giving a very red and excoriated (burning) appearance. Moisture damage in effect gives pressure damage a head start, so it is vital that adequate pressure relief be provided. Moisture lesions are often mistaken for pressure ulcers, but Table 42.1 details the subtle differences between the two types of skin trauma.

A moisture lesion or a pressure ulcer?

The differences between moisture lesions and pressure ulcers are given in Table 42.1.

Prevention and management of moisture lesions

As always, prevention is much better than cure; therefore, to begin with, as far as possible, it is vital to address the cause of the incontinence (or sweating, or both). This may include instigating a regular toileting regimen (e.g. two or three times hourly) and excellence in skin care in case of incontinence. In any event, it is essential that expert advice be sought from a continence specialist nurse who is able to assess, treat and manage the cause of incontinence.

In the meantime, in addition to the preceding points, it is crucial that the following care be taken in order to avoid moisture lesions:

1 The application of appropriate-sized continence pads; these must be fitted to the conformity of the body and should not be placed as a sheet under the patient. Modern pads have an indicator when they need changing (e.g. a line that appears on the outer pad). Choosing the right sized pad will mean that maximum wear time and cost-effectiveness will be achieved; the pad will be changed before it reaches its maximum absorbency, after which the moisture will sit against the skin. It is therefore important to look for the indicator line. However, this method of capturing moisture must not be a substitute for toilet opportunities.
2 The use of an appropriate moisture barrier cream that assists in preventing moisture sitting next to the skin. It is important to be aware of the variety of products on the market, and following expert advice can help with this. Many barrier products are difficult to spread onto the skin due to the consistency; applying and washing off the barrier cream can cause skin trauma. Furthermore, some barrier creams (e.g. Sudocrem) are contraindicated for use with continence pads, as this product (as well as others) can 'clog' the pores of the pad, thereby preventing moisture soaking into the pad. This results in moisture sitting against the skin, which eventually penetrates the cream, causing moisture damage. It is therefore advisable to use tissue viability recommended barrier creams, such as Cavilon cream.
3 Once there are breaks in the skin caused by moisture (and/or pressure ulcers), it is advisable to stop the use of creams and use a barrier spray instead (e.g. Cavilon spray). This creates a 'protective film' that moisture is unable to penetrate. Applying creams to moisture lesions simply adds to the moisture levels, which encourage further bacterial growth, thereby increasing the risk of cellulitis.
4 Keep skin clean and dry using a moisturising barrier cream (e.g. Cavilon cream), as already stated. Avoid the use of alcohol wipes and soaps to wash the skin; use wash creams instead (e.g. Tena wash cream). Soaps containing alcohol cause the skin to dry and crack, and, when urine or faecal matter get on to the skin, it causes a stinging sensation and increases the risk of infection.
5 Ensure adequate nutrition and hydration. A good, well-balanced diet and around 2 litres of fluids daily maintain maximum skin integrity.
6 If the patient is unable to reposition himself/herself independently in response to pressure, it is vital that care be provided to ensure that regular repositioning is carried out in order to prevent pressure ulcers. Moisture lesions can give pressure damage a 'head start', and they can quickly deteriorate to deeper tissue damage.

43 Surgical wounds

Table 43.1 Description of types of surgical wounds.

Type of surgical wound	Description
Clean	An uninfected operative wound in which no inflammation is encountered and in which the respiratory tract, alimentary, genital or uninfected urinary tracts are not entered
Clean-contaminated	Operative wounds in which the respiratory, alimentary, genital or urinary tract is entered under controlled conditions and without unusual contamination
Contaminated	Open, fresh or accidental wounds; operations with major breaks in sterile technique or gross spillage from the gastrointestinal tract; and incisions in which acute, non-purulent inflammation is encountered
Dirty or infected	Old traumatic wounds with retained devitalised tissue, and those that involve existing clinical infection

Figure 43.1 A surgical adhesive strip.

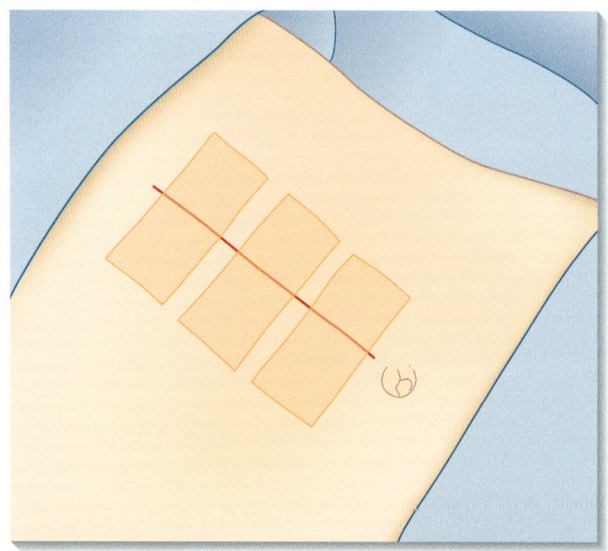

Figure 43.2 Paper strip dressing.

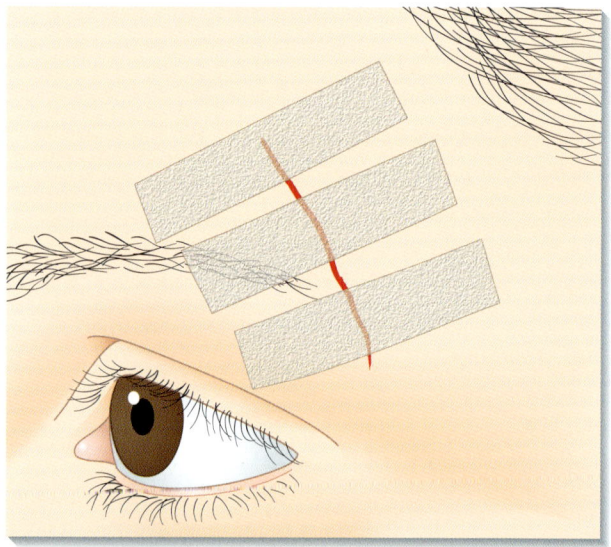

Figure 43.3 Staples.

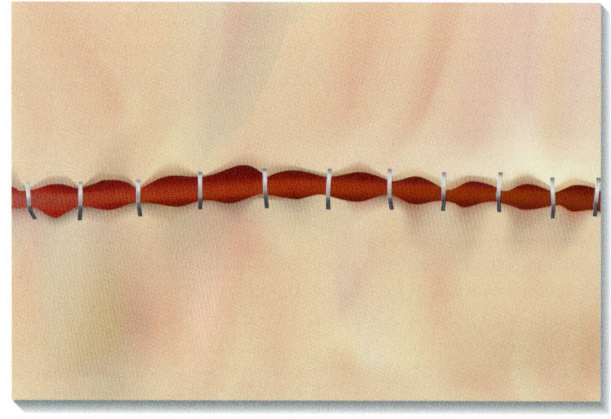

Figure 43.4 Sutures.

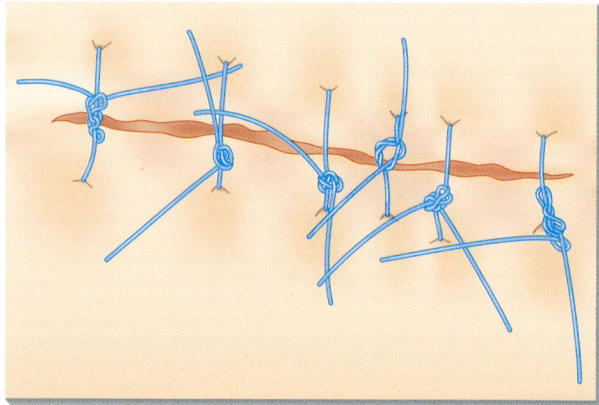

Source: P. Vong. Reproduced with permission of P. Vong.

Wound Care at a Glance, Second Edition. Ian Peate and Melanie Stephens.
© 2020 John Wiley & Sons Ltd. Published 2020 by John Wiley & Sons Ltd.
Companion website: http://www.ataglanceseries.com/nursing/woundcare/

Most surgical wounds are closed at the time of surgery with the wound edges held together with mechanical aids, such as sutures, staples (clips), paper strips or glue, or a combination of these. This type of closure is known as *primary intention*. As a result, the wound has a minimal exposed surface area with very little tissue loss and in most cases the wound heals fully within 3–4 weeks, as it follows the healing process, which has been described in earlier chapters. However, on occasions, the wound dehisces (i.e. bursts open) for a variety of reasons, and requires healing by secondary intention, which means that it requires appropriate dressings to create an optimum environment to encourage it through the healing process. Postoperative wounds can be classified using the 1964 National Academy of Science categories as either clean, clean-contaminated, contaminated and dirty infection (NICE, 2019, p. 9; see Table 43.1).

To prevent and treat surgical site infection and complications, some guidelines have been developed to provide a structured approach to preoperative, intraoperative and postoperative care.

Preoperative care

Patients at risk of postoperative surgical site infection or complications should be identified preoperatively. Interprofessional teams should explore the potential benefits and risks of preoperative bathing, washing and hair removal.

Intraoperative care

The surgical team must ensure that they adhere to personal and protective equipment and procedures intraoperatively, such as the wearing of theatre clothes, gowns and masks. Drapes may be used over the patient. Handwashing prior to the commencement of the surgical procedure should include the use of correct solutions and technique (surgical hand preparation). Suitable skin preparation solutions and aseptic technique should be used: prior to the first incision, during the operation and postoperatively. Consideration must also be given to ensuring that the patient is kept normothermic during the procedure, and, if necessary, warming blankets must be used preoperatively, intraoperatively and postoperatively. Deliberation should be given to the most appropriate topical intrawound solutions and antibiotics, suturing materials, wound closure techniques and dressings used to cover the wound post-procedure. The dressing should be left undisturbed for the first 48 hours, provided no adverse events occur in the meantime (such as wound pain, pyrexia or wound discharge).

Postoperative care

The postoperative complications include bleeding and wound infection. In order to try and reduce these complications, NICE guidance suggests that the surgical team consider the use of postoperative drains, antibiotics, dressings, wound-cleansing techniques and debridement for wounds healing by secondary intention. Each patient should be assessed on a case-by-case holistic assessment to decide on the appropriate course of action.

Complicated surgical wounds

Bleeding

In the event of bleeding, it is vital that this be arrested by using firm pressure, applying alginates that contain haemostatic properties (e.g. Kaltostat) directly to the wound. If not arrested within 20 minutes, it is vital that the patient be referred to a senior health care professional such as a doctor without delay.

Infection

At least 5% of patients undergoing a surgical procedure develop a surgical site infection that may become evident within 7–10 days post-operation (NICE 2019). Postoperatively, an interactive (insulating) dressing must be applied to the surgical wound. In most cases, the dressing is best left undisturbed for the first 48 hours, after which it should be removed to observe for signs of infection and dehiscence. If the dressing becomes saturated with wound exudate, if bleeding is observed, if there is a sudden increase in pain or if a malodour is noted, then the dressing should be removed for observation and wound assessment. Dressing replacement should be applied by use of the 'aseptic non-touch technique'.

Fistula

A fistula is a passage between two organs, with common ones forming between the bowel and skin. Patients usually have a malignancy or inflammatory bowel disease.

Wound dehiscence

There are several reasons why a wound becomes dehisced, for example, swelling caused by the trauma of the surgical procedure; obesity; excessive tissue loss causing greater tension on the wound closure; and infection or underlying abscess formation. Each of these put too much tension on the mechanical aids used to close the wound, thereby causing the wound to dehisce. Many cases of dehiscence are unavoidable, but with good wound management these wounds will usually heal well by secondary intention. However, wounds that heal this way tend to have larger scars, which may be weaker in tensile strength than the previous tissues and may have a poorer cosmetic result than a scar that has healed by primary intention.

Cavity

A surgical wound that is dehisced may become a cavity wound, depending on how deep it dehisces, and the layers of the skin and subcutaneous tissues get involved to become a cavity wound.

Evisceration

Nearly 30% of all surgical wounds result in evisceration. This is when the gastrointestinal tract protrudes the wound opening. This is very frightening for the patient and considered a medical emergency. The patient should be assessed for signs of shock, and moist dressing must be applied to the open wound and bowel. The foot of the bed should be elevated by 20°, and medical advice should be sought instantly. Patients often return to theatre for further surgery and insertion of Teflon grafts. The wound may be left open to heal by secondary intention, and negative wound therapy or wound mangers may be used.

Documenting a surgical wound

Although it is anticipated that most surgical wounds heal spontaneously and require little intervention, it is essential that at least the wound site, size and wound closure aids are documented, to begin with. On first review or dressing change (whichever is sooner) of the wound, the nurse should record the condition of the surrounding skin and suture line as a baseline condition. In the event of dehiscence, the wound ought to be fully assessed and the findings documented on a wound assessment chart (see Figure 20.1).

Wound irrigation

If the wound requires irrigation (i.e. usually when there is any loose debris or excess exudate), warm sterile saline should be used during the first 48 hours post-operation. However, this wound cleansing practice depends on the location of the wound on the body, and on local infection control and wound care policies. Some patients with wounds in their hair or perineal area may have their wounds left undressed and cleansed with warm water, as currently there is no conclusive evidence with regard to wound complications of early or delayed postoperative showering or bathing.

Removal of sutures, staples, paper strips and adhesive

- *Adhesive* (Figure 43.1): It is not necessary to remove adhesives from wounds; they should be left to auto-debride from the wound.
- *Paper strips* (Figure 43.2): Must be kept dry until they are due for removal in around 7 days. It is advisable to soak the strips before removal; lift the strip from both outer edges towards the suture line, then gently remove them from the wound. If a wound dehisces, it is not necessary to reapply strips to hold the edges together and secondary intention healing should be applied.
- *Staples* (Figure 43.3): It is not necessary to cleanse the wound before or after staple removal. Staples are usually removed in 7–10 days unless specified otherwise. Special disposable staple removers are used to remove the staples.
- *Sutures* (Figure 43.4): It is not necessary to cleanse the wound. There are two types of sutures; removable and dissolvable. Removable sutures are usually black or navy blue in colour and are usually removed in 7–10 days post-operation, unless specified otherwise. The suture can be one long subcutaneous stitch or can be individual. It is important for the nurse to determine the number and type of sutures used before removal, in order to ensure that the correct care can be provided. Dissolvable sutures are usually flesh (pale pink) or violet in colour. This type of suture does not require removal and gets dissolved when in contact with subcutaneous exudate in around 60–71 days.

Once mechanical aids are removed, it is essential that the wound continues to be observed for any signs of dehiscence and infection, and, over time, for abnormal scar tissue formation, each of which requires referral for appropriate intervention.

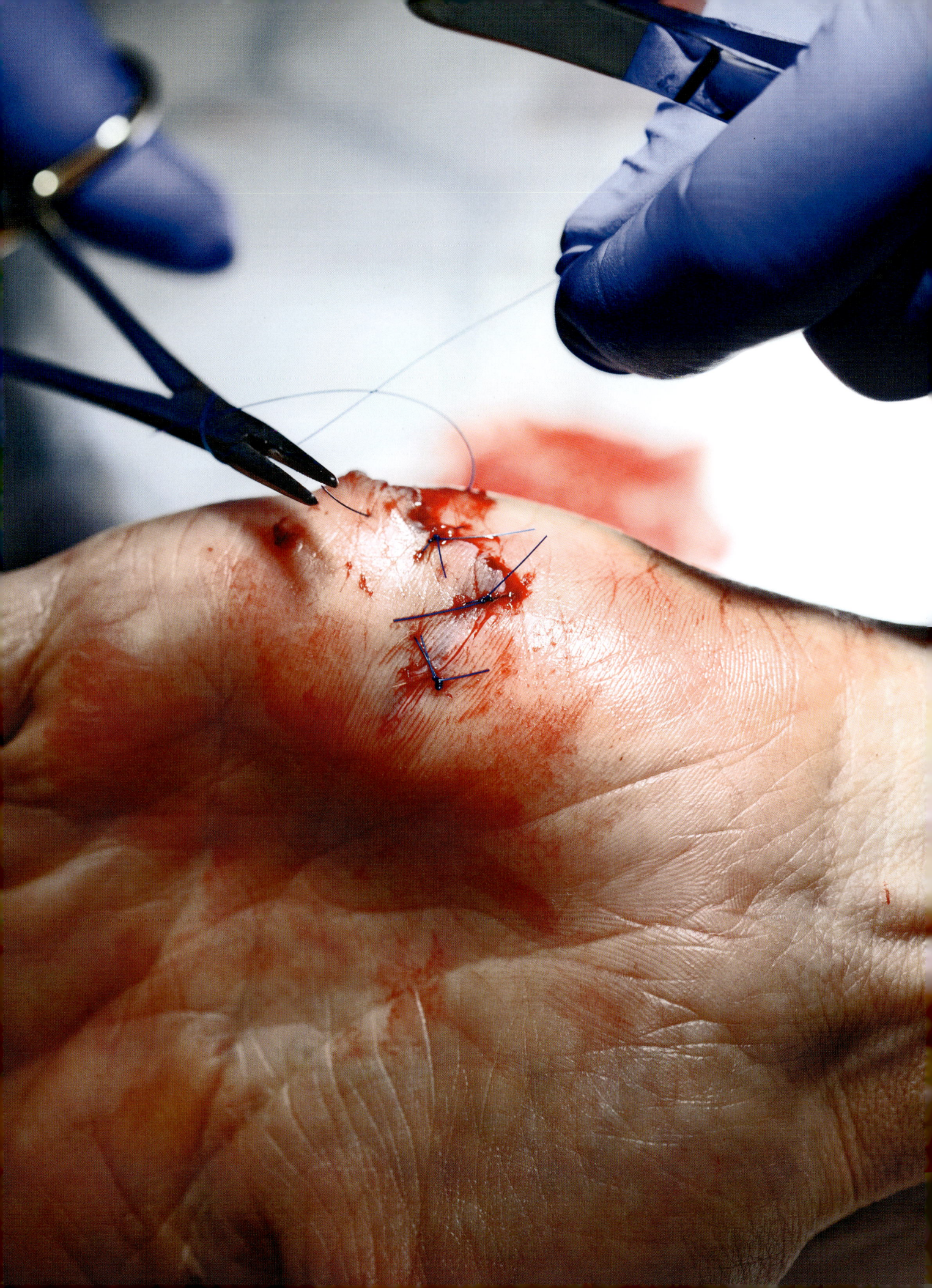

44 Traumatic wounds

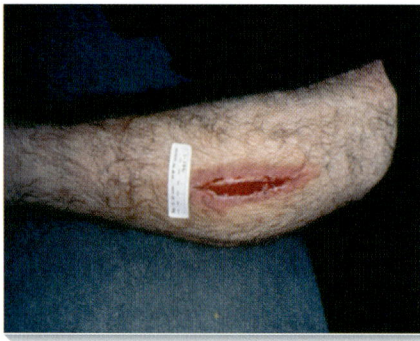

Figure 44.1 Incision/cut.

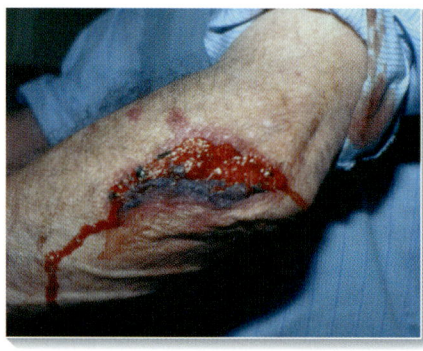

Figure 44.2 Laceration.

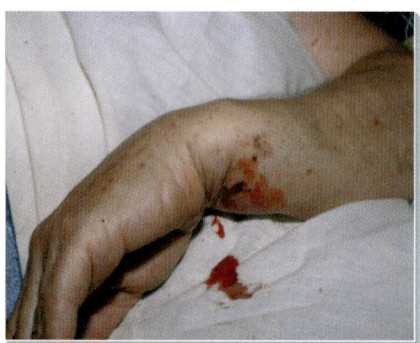

Figure 44.3 Puncture wound.

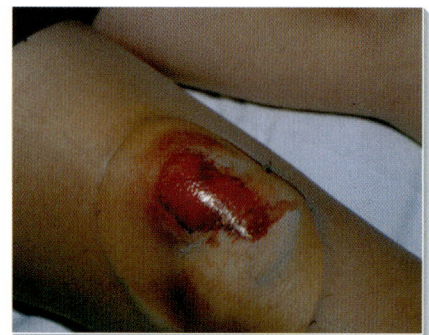

Figure 44.4 Abrasion/friction.

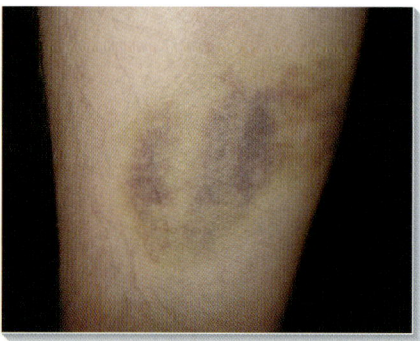

Figure 44.5 Contusion/bruise.

Table 44.1 International Skin Tear Advisory Panel (ISTAP) Skin Tear Classification System.

Skin tear classification	Type 1: No skin loss	Type 2: Partial flap loss	Type 3: Total flap loss
Description of skin loss	Skin tear that is either a straight line or a flap that can be repositioned over the wound bed	Skin tear that is a partial flap that cannot be repositioned over the wound bed	Total flap loss to whole of the wound bed

Wound Care at a Glance, Second Edition. Ian Peate and Melanie Stephens.
© 2020 John Wiley & Sons Ltd. Published 2020 by John Wiley & Sons Ltd.
Companion website: http://www.ataglanceseries.com/nursing/woundcare/

Traumatic wounds are caused by a sudden or unplanned external insult. There are many types of traumatic wounds, which may include injuries from road traffic accidents, gunshot wounds, domestic accidents, trips and falls and burns from heat, cold, electricity and chemicals.

The principles of wound healing should be applied in all cases; however, many traumatic wounds require thorough irrigation and/or debridement both initially and ongoing through the wound-healing process, as required. It is essential that the wound is protected from further trauma, and the choice of dressing can go some way to achieve this. As with any wound, the underlying cause of the wound must be identified and either eliminated or controlled in order to avoid recurrence of the injury; for example, if an individual spills a hot drink on a regular basis, action must be taken to avoid such spillages (e.g. reducing the heat of the drink). The following descriptions are of common types of wounds caused by trauma. A brief outline of each is presented in the following text.

Incision (cut) (Figure 44.1): Usually caused by a 'slice' to the skin and underlying tissues by a sharp-edged thing, a shard of glass, scalpel, knife or a sheet of metal. The edges are usually clearly defined with little, if any, tissue loss. The edges of the wound can be held together without undue tension by mechanical aides (e.g. clips, sutures, strips, adhesive or a combination of these). As these wounds heal by primary intention, they require minimal wound care after closure. A hydrofibre and a film dressing are the appropriate dressings that promote healing and allow absorption of exudate, which is usually minimal in these wound types.

Laceration (Figure 44.2): Usually caused by a blow from a blunt object, causing the skin to split/tear into a skin flap, particularly over a bony prominence. A common example of this type of wound is the pretibial laceration. The skin flap can be thick or thin depending on the extent of the tissue destruction. There is often some skin/tissue loss noted, and often the edges do not meet due to surrounding swelling caused by the injury. Where little or no swelling occurs, the wound can often be healed by primary intention. If there is any tissue loss or extensive swelling, the wound must heal by secondary intention. Often, a combination of wound closure is required. In either type of closure, it is vital that this wound be thoroughly irrigated to remove loose debris, and the flap edges should be rolled back in order to allow epithelial to epithelial tissue repair. The mechanism of injury indicates if the tissues are likely to swell, which assists with the decision-making process regarding choice of wound closure. A hydrofibre and a film dressing are the appropriate dressings, which promote healing, allowing the absorption of exudate, which is usually minimal in these wound types.

Skin tear: This injury is usually caused by the skin being: torn by a sharp object, such as a nail, or a fingernail and/or shear and friction forces separating the epidermis from the dermis or dermis from the subcutaneous layers. Skin tears are commonly associated with elderly patients because of fragility of the skin from long-term side effects of medication, age and altered skin function. Skin tears can be regarded as a laceration and wound closure is determined by the amount of tissue loss, if any as with lacerations. It is vital that the wound is thoroughly irrigated before closure to evacuate debris from the wound, in order to reduce the risk of infection. Skin tears should not be misdiagnosed as pressure ulcers and should be classified using the ISTAP system (see Table 44.1). The treatment and management of skin tears should be based upon the preservation of any skin flaps, maintenance of surrounding tissue, reduction of risk for infection and prevention of further trauma.

Puncture/penetrating (Figure 44.3): These wounds are caused by a sharp, pointed element penetrating into deep tissues, or by a bone fracture piercing through the skin and underlying tissues (as seen in Figure 44.3), a bullet wound or a bite (animal, human or insect). On removal of the causing element, the puncture wound may appear small and insignificant, but should not be underestimated; damage to underlying structures is highly probable with this type of wound (e.g. tendon, internal organs, nerves, blood vessels), as is the risk of infection. It is vital that these wounds are thoroughly explored by an appropriate health care practitioner and/or X-rayed to ensure that there is no remaining foreign body or underlying trauma before the wound entry site is closed. Often, antibiotics are given in high-risk injuries, such as bites (particularly punctures caused by a cat bite).

Burn/scald: It can be caused by heat, cold, electricity or chemicals; it is vital that the cause of the burn be identified before treating, such as:

- *Heat*: Wounds ought to be cooled by using cold running water.
- *Cold*: Burns (often called 'frostbite') must not be warmed up but protected with a clean towel to prevent further heat loss.
- *Electricity*: First and foremost, the rescuer must ensure his/her own safety and should switch off the electric supply before attending to the patient. The patient needs to be admitted to the emergency department to check for cardiac function, as the electricity can cause internal burns and affect heart rhythms.

Abrasion/friction (Figure 44.4): This is a wound that results in superficial dermal loss, but friction can cause deep abrasions, depending on the mechanism of injury, and indeed can result in full-thickness tissue loss. The skin is generally subject to low levels of friction on a daily basis, which may cause thinning of the dead epithelial layers initially but could traumatise the protective cuboidal cells (the living layer of the epidermis), resulting in an open wound. Common areas that are affected with friction are the heels and elbow. In areas at risk, a film dressing can be applied, which can offer protection to vulnerable areas; and, in the event of trauma, hydrofibre and a film dressing would be an appropriate dressing, which promotes healing by allowing the absorption of exudate, which is usually minimal in these types of wounds.

Contusion/bruising (Figure 44.5): This occurs due to trauma against tissues, causing a rupture to a blood vessel(s) that allows blood to seep out into the surrounding tissues, causing a haematoma. It is important to arrest the bleeding to reduce the size of the haematoma. Initially, the bleeding produces a 'red' and often swollen appearance to the skin, and, as the underlying wound ages, the deoxygenated blood darkens, causing discolouration commonly called a 'bruise'. It is therefore regarded as a 'closed wound'. A contusion may be present around other types of wounds caused at the time of the injury, and commonly presents with a laceration due to the extensive effect of the blunt trauma affecting wider tissues. If there is no breach to the skin around the contusion, then no specific dressing is required, and the venous return and lymphatic drainage eventually disperse the haematoma, which resolves usually within 10–14 days.

Avulsions: These occur when the skin is pulled off with or without the involvement of bone by objects such as doors, machinery or personal/household items (rings, curtain rings). An avulsion often occurs on the patient's fingers and toes; but, in manufacturing-type jobs, injuries can include avulsion of a partial or whole limb.

Bites: Human or animal bites sometimes result in wounds. These wounds are heavily contaminated with bacteria and necessitate initial assessment for the type of bacteria and any toxins which may be present. Bite wounds require thorough cleansing and heal via tertiary intention.

45 Burns and scalds

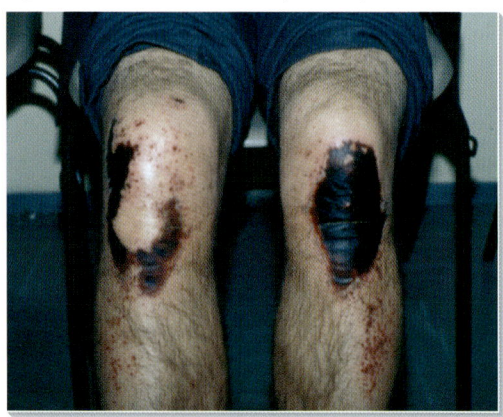

Figure 45.1 Chemical burn (cement).

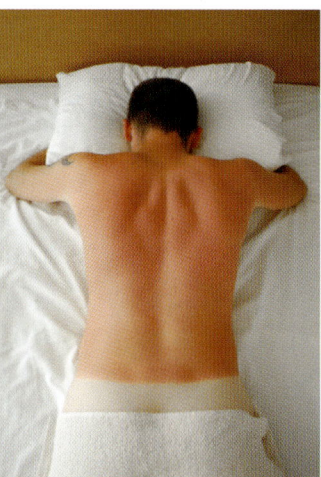

Figure 45.3 Sunburn.

Figure 45.2 Body map showing the rule of nines.

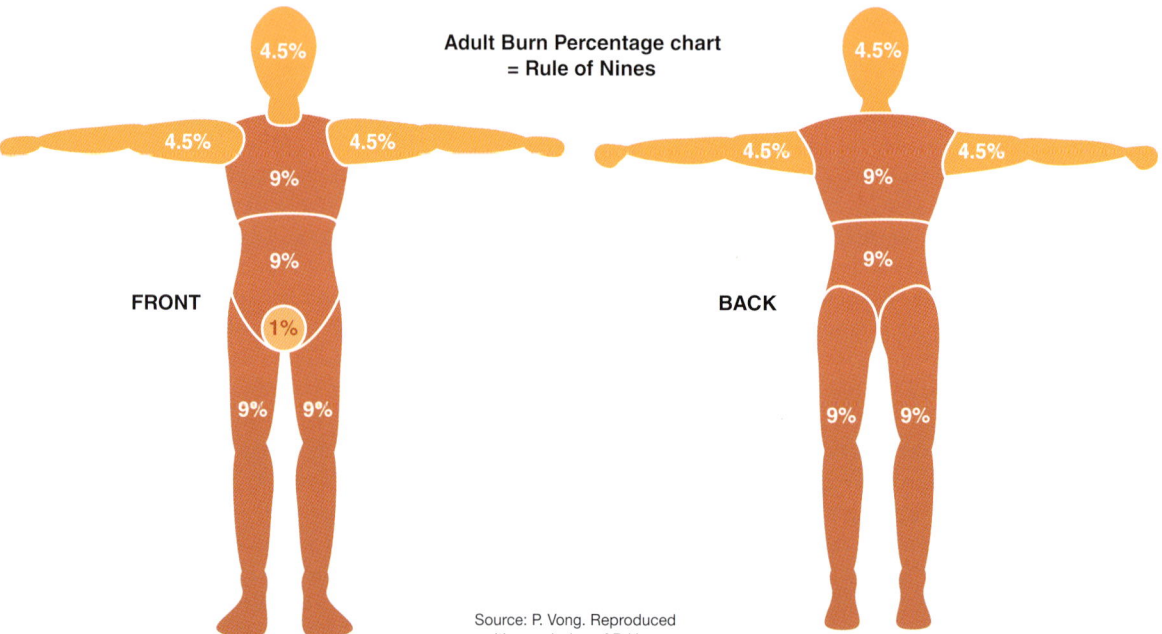

Adult Burn Percentage chart = Rule of Nines

Source: P. Vong. Reproduced with permission of P. Vong.

Table 45.1 Estimated total body surface area calculated using the rule of nines.

Anatomical area	% Total body surface area
Head/neck	9
Each arm	9
Anterior thorax	18
Posterior thorax	18
Each leg	18
Perineum	1

Table 45.2 Features of varying depths of burns.

Superficial partial thickness of the epidermis	Red but without blistering. Not usually life threatening; no scarring
Superficial dermal	May have small blistering and/or total epidermal loss. The area is usually wet due to loss of interstitial fluid. Usually has minimal scarring. Blanches (goes white) when pressed
Deep dermal	Total epidermal loss or blistering, red in appearance, does not blanch when pressed and there is loss of sensation. Scarring is likely

Wound Care at a Glance, Second Edition. Ian Peate and Melanie Stephens.
© 2020 John Wiley & Sons Ltd. Published 2020 by John Wiley & Sons Ltd.
Companion website: http://www.ataglanceseries.com/nursing/woundcare/

The origin of tissue destruction by burns and scalds must be identified, as each type of trauma requires different management strategies. Scalds are caused by hot liquids or steam and burns are caused by hot or cold objects, fire, chemicals (Figure 45.1) or electricity. This chapter will focus on the long-term management of each type of burn/scald.

Assessment and resuscitation

First and foremost, it is vital that an assessment of the burns and total surface area affected be established, and resuscitation applied as necessary, depending on the total body surface area (TBSA) affected. In the UK, burns with severity greater than 10% TBSA in children and 15% TBSA in adults requires intravenous fluid infusion; burns with greater than 30% TBSA could prove fatal. In children, these percentages are much less, and any burn/scald affecting even just 5% requires hospitalisation. Table 45.1 represents the estimated TBSA in adults using the rule of nines (Figure 45.2), a commonly used method in the UK to estimate the extent of burns.

Severity

The severity of a burn is determined by the surface area and the depth of the affected injury. The depths of different types of burns are described in Table 45.2.

Burns or scalds that are circumferential or affecting moveable areas, such as the palm of hands, over joints and on the face, require medical attention irrespective of size, as the maturative phase of wound healing can lead to contractures, thereby limiting movement and/or causing deformities. The greatest risk to patients with burns is infection due to the skin's breach over a large area; therefore, aseptic technique when dealing with burns/scalds is paramount. Silver antimicrobial dressings are commonly used on burns (e.g. silver sulphadiazine cream, Aquacel Ag) in order to provide the patient with a protective barrier.

Management of burns

Minor burns (Figure 45.3): First aid includes cooling the burn, covering the burn and relieving the pain.

- *Cooling the burn*: Reducing the heat by running under tepid water. This is optimum if commenced within 20 minutes of the injury and continued for 30 minutes.
- *Covering the burn*: In 'cling-film', covered by a towel.
- *Relieving the pain*: Cooling and covering the burn aids in pain reduction; however, some patients require a combination of paracetamol and non-steroidal anti-inflammatory or low-dose opioid. Wound management depends upon the severity of the burn and may include soothing gels or creams to dressings based upon assessment of the level of exudate, risk of infection and adherence of dressing to the wound bed.

Major burns: First aid may include upper airway management, so immediate medical help must be called for. Prevent further fluid loss by wrapping the burns in cling-film; keep the patient warm to reduce their risk of hypothermia, as they will have lost their ability to control body temperature due to excess skin loss. *Do not* apply cold water or ice to the burns, as this causes hypothermia. These patients should be referred immediately to a specialist burn unit as soon as they are medically resuscitated and stabilised.

Chemical burns (Figure 45.1): Irrigate the affected area for a long period using large amounts of water; sometimes this can be for as long as 10 hours in cases of alkali burns (e.g. cement). Using a urine dipstick against the wet skin over the burn can identify if irrigation is sufficient (when a normal pH of 5.5 is achieved). Irrigation may be necessary for longer periods, particularly if the eye is affected.

Electrical burns: These often present as small entry and exit wounds, concealing the true extent of the damage caused. Tissue necrosis and gangrene can occur, and the patient should be monitored for ventricular fibrillation and cardiac arrest.

Referral to a specialist burn unit

In many cases, the patient requires the medical attention of a specialist burn unit, and it is vital that the patient suffering from any of the following burns be transferred to the unit without delay. The patient must be immediately medically resuscitated and stabilised for transfer. The following list is not exhaustive, and any patient with an uncertain wound must be referred to a burn unit for specialist advice:

- Any child under the age of 10 years or an adult over the age of 49 years who has sustained a severe burn must be transferred to a specialist unit without delay.
- Patients with circumferential burns.
- Those with burns to their face, hands, over joints or on the perineum.
- Any electrical burns.
- Chemical burns affecting 5% of the body surface area.
- Any patient with exposure to chemicals or radiation.
- Any patient with underlying medical conditions/comorbidities.
- Pregnant women.
- Large affected areas (5% for the under-16 age group, and 10% for the over-16 age group).
- All full-thickness burns (any age group, any extent).
- Suspected inhalation injury.
- Associated injuries (such as fractures, head injuries, crush injuries).
- Septic burn wounds.

46 Atypical wounds

Figure 46.1 Bullous pemphigoid.

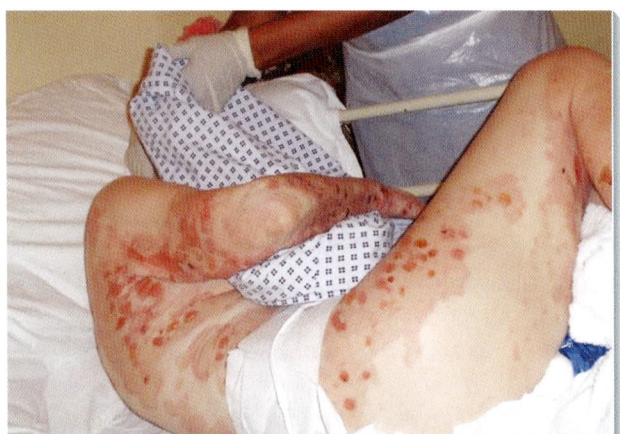

Figure 46.2 Cutaneous TB under the tongue.

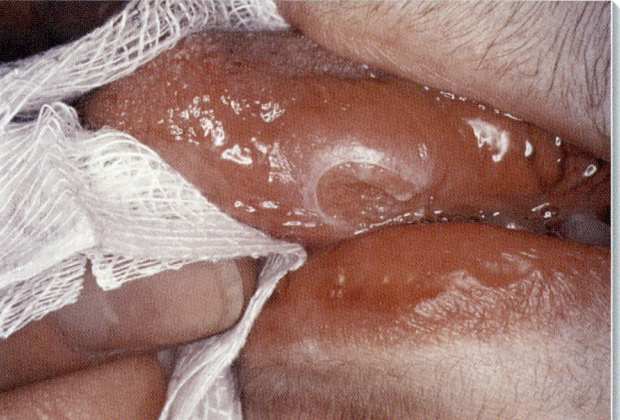

Source: CDC Public Health Image Library.

Wound Care at a Glance, Second Edition. Ian Peate and Melanie Stephens.
© 2020 John Wiley & Sons Ltd. Published 2020 by John Wiley & Sons Ltd.
Companion website: http://www.ataglanceseries.com/nursing/woundcare/

Atypical wounds

Atypical wounds are those that are of unknown origin, or those that present in unusual sites and with abnormal presentation. It is thought that many of these wound types are caused by conditions such as malignancy and rare illnesses. They tend to fall into the causation categories of inflammatory wounds, autoimmune disease, infective wounds, external cause or genetic/hereditary causes. This chapter will consider the most common types of atypical wounds that the average nurse is likely to encounter in his/her nursing career.

Bullous pemphigoid (Figure 46.1): This is a rare autoimmune condition that generally affects the elderly population. It occurs when the immune system forms antibodies that then attack its own tissues. Blisters occur that can become painful; as this is an autoimmune disease, it renders the patient at increased risk of infection via these skin breaches along the dermis/epidermis junction. On occasions, these blisters present in the mouth, throat and the intestinal tract; these can also occur in the trachea, and this is a life-threatening situation that requires immediate hospital admission for mechanical ventilation. The mainstay treatment for this condition is steroids. The priority of the wound treatment is to protect the patient from infection as far as possible, by using antimicrobial dressings that also provide a moist environment in order to prevent adherence and pain.

Pyoderma gangrenosum: This is a rare condition that causes skin ulceration and inflammation for unknown reasons. It can often be found in traumatic wounds, particularly in those patients who may unknowingly have this condition. The lesions usually occur as red, elevated eruptions that resemble insect bites and can be very painful. Its treatment is similar to the treatment of any other wound type, but may include the application of topical steroids, following the advice of a specialist dermatologist.

Blastomycosis: This is a rare infection caused by inhaling fungi from soil, wood or plants. It can cause skin lesions and is associated with breathing difficulties and by bone and joint pain.

Cutaneous tuberculosis (Figure 46.2): This is caused by the invasion of the same bacteria that causes pulmonary tuberculosis. The skin lesions present as purple or red/brownish watery growths and commonly affect the limbs and buttocks. The lesions may persist for years and can clear up without any active treatment; however, some lead to limb amputations. Its treatment is usually with antibiotics and topical antimicrobials that may be required for several months or years.

Scleroderma: This is a chronic autoimmune condition that presents inflammation and tissue fibrosis (skin hardening and tightening), discolouration and itching. It can be very painful, especially as the skin hardens.

There are many other less common atypical wounds; however, in most cases, the principles of wound healing are applied in order to promote healing, prevent or eliminate infection and to prevent trauma. Therefore, the use of non-adherent antimicrobial dressings and specialist advice on the treatments of the underlying causes (once diagnosed) must be adhered to. If in doubt, the patient must be referred to a member of the dermatology or tissue viability team.

One very common atypical wound condition that most nurses find difficult to deal with is that of hypergranulation. It is therefore important to discuss this in this section, although it could be regarded as a normal, although unwanted, aspect of wound healing.

Hypergranulation (over granulation): A wound of any type can appear to progress towards healing very nicely until such time that it begins to over granulate; then the progression to healing appears to stop. Occasionally, it proceeds without intervention, but often, it does not progress until the wound environment is altered from moist to dry. Hypergranulation commonly occurs around drain sites (e.g. suprapubic catheters and PEG sites) and can be problematic for the nurse and painful for the patient. The cause of hypergranulation is important to understand, so that it can be avoided and/or treated in a timely fashion.

- *Appearance*: Hypergranulation appears like a healthy but raised/swollen granulation tissue that often sits proud to the surrounding skin level. The term 'hypergranulation' suggests that there are more granulation cells growing than are usually expected; however, this is incorrect.
- *The cause*: This situation is thought to result from high levels of bacteria, the waste products of which alter the pH levels on the wound bed, which then traumatises the granulation cells, preventing them from maturing and 'shrinking' to their normal size. Their appearance for this phenomenon is larger than would otherwise be. Once this situation occurs, it is difficult for the wound to progress to healing until the condition of the wound is altered to reduce bacterial levels, which in turn regulates the pH levels on the wound bed; any granulation cells that are produced continue to remain swollen, and epithelial cells are reluctant to migrate across the altered pH levels of the wound until rectified. In order to rectify the wound conditions and to allow maturation of the granulation cells and migration of epithelial cells, there are two options available: (i) absorbing all of the moisture from the wound to dry out the wound bed, using absorbent dressing; this changes the environment the bacteria have become familiar with, and so they die. Once the wound is dry, the granulation cells become mature and shrink, and moist wound healing can then be reintroduced, so that healing can be promoted; and (ii) the application of an antimicrobial dressing (ideally one that does not achieve a moist environment – e.g. Actisorb Silver or Acticoat) which kills the bacteria causing the problem, covered by a foam dressing to absorb moisture. Once the situation is rectified and a dry environment is achieved, the hypergranulation tissue reduces in size and healing progresses as normal, so that moist wound healing can resume. In the event of a rise in exudate levels, the nurse must be alert to the recurrence of this situation, as bacterial levels increase once again; thus, repeat interventions are required until resolved once again.

Treatment and prevention: Atypical wounds can be extremely challenging to treat, as they frequently necessitate referral to a team of specialists/doctors from different disciplines. These wounds are diagnosed by a medical officer reviewing the patient's medical, family and social history, completing a physical examination of the patient and his/her wound(s). A discussion about the patient's hobbies, recreational activities, holidays and exposure to harmful substances must be conducted. Tests to aid diagnosis of an atypical wound include tissue biopsy, blood tests, X-ray, CT scan and MRI scan.

Care plans and management should include: Categorising the causative agent(s) of the wound; treating or eradicating the underlying cause with surgery, chemotherapy, radiotherapy or antibiotics; appropriate wound care; pain management; review of the patient's lifestyle choices; attention to general health and well-being; psychological therapy; and correct medication.

47 Wounds in different populations

Figure 47.1 Homelessness.

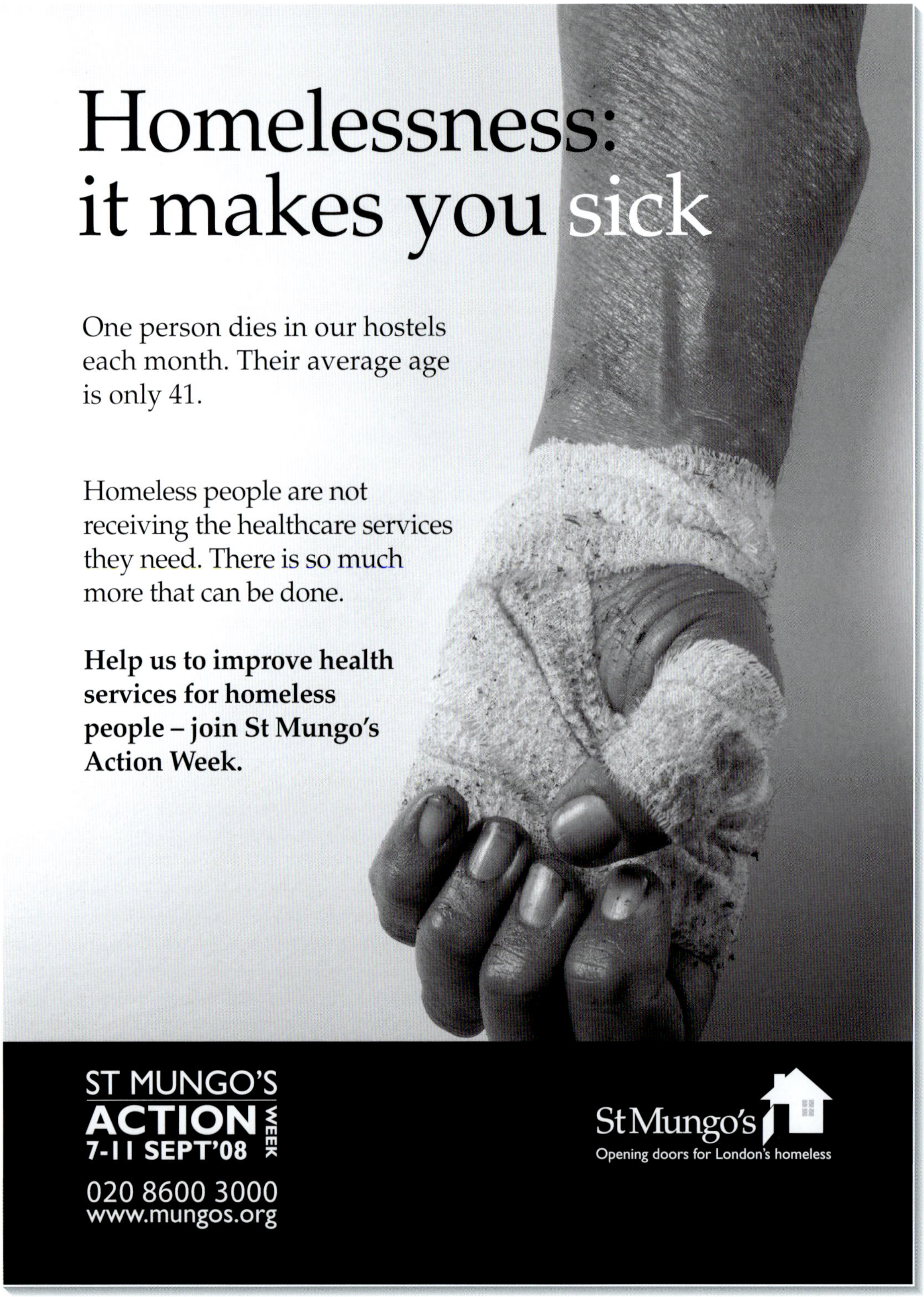

Source: St Mungo's 2019. Seeking permission to reproduce.

Hard to reach, seldom heard

There are members of our community who are often said to be 'hard-to-reach' through traditional healthcare services; they are sometimes referred to as:

- Seldom heard
- Socially excluded
- Easy to ignore
- Hidden populations.

Commissioners and providers of wound care services and other statutory and voluntary organisations working with hard-to-reach groups such as St Mungo's can achieve better outcomes through targeted action to identify at-risk patients early and providing intensive clinical and social support to help them (see Figure 47.1).

Traditional hospital and primary care services are not always the best way of reaching and treating some groups of people, and services can be hard to access for some vulnerable people. People who are hardest to reach can include:

- Those with drug or alcohol addiction.
- Asylum seekers and refugees.
- Homeless and insecurely housed people.
- Gypsies and travellers.
- Those within the criminal justice system.
- People with learning disabilities.
- People with long-term mental health problems.

Older people and those with mental health illness or learning disabilities have worse health experiences than the rest of the population. Accessing primary and secondary care differs amongst populations, as does the quality of some of these services; this, in turn, has an impact on health outcomes.

The homeless, drug users, migrants and those in places of detention (including prisons) are not homogeneous groups; it is acknowledged that many of them are difficult to contact. There are certain groups who are particularly 'hard-to-reach' and highly mobile. Society has a tendency to marginalise, isolate and socially exclude some groups. They are not often in contact with any statutory and, in some instances, voluntary services; they may be unaware of, or may choose not to access, such services.

These people may find it difficult to recognise the problems with their wounds and to access diagnostic and treatment services. They may also have problems in self-care and attending regular appointments for clinical follow-up. This can lead to incomplete treatment with serious consequences.

Homeless and insecurely housed people

Accessing healthcare is often problematic for homeless people, due to difficulties in registering with a GP, problematic appointment systems, lack of access to a phone or transport and disordered lifestyles, and some may have experienced discriminatory attitudes by healthcare providers.

People who are homeless have rates of physical ill health many times greater than those of the general population. Addressing and treating their health needs can be challenging, sometimes due to missed appointments, comorbidities, lack of concordance and poor nutrition.

Factors that increase homeless people's risk for acute and chronic wounds include communal living and eating, lack of facilities for washing and toileting, unsafe and unsanitary shelters, exposure to crime and trauma, inadequate nutrition, no place for bed rest, no place to keep medications, excessive smoking and drinking, little or no income and absence of family and other support to help in times of illness. Substance abuse and mental illnesses may affect a person's ability to understand and follow a wound care treatment plan.

These factors are associated with the homeless person, the service and the practitioner:

- Concordance and 'buy in' from the patient, attendance at clinic, assessment, diagnosis and treatment.
- A non-judgmental approach and good relationships.
- Clinic accessibility.
- Prescribing and accessibility to specialist wound care products that meet the needs of the person's life style.
- Effective multidisciplinary working with the community.
- Consideration and treatment of comorbidities.
- Provision or referral to other services.

The Queen's Nursing Institute has provided a resource that can help nurses assess, for example, the healthcare needs of those people who are homeless. The template within the resource offers guidance and support to nurses.

The therapeutic relationship

The value of a good rapport with patients is sometimes underestimated. Most service providers are clearly health focused. There is also a need for value service delivery in a framework of general social support, advocacy, assisting and non-judgmental care.

Relationships with service providers are often valued more than treatment options or therapies provided; it is important to attend to this basic human need first. The therapeutic relationship is one that offers respect, trust and care to the other.

A relationship that conveys acceptance and support to patients may reduce levels of cortisol that is often elevated when a person is anxious or has concerns about health. Raised cortisol levels have an impact on wound healing; practitioners should adopt actions to minimise stress, and in so doing the healing response is likely to improve.

Homeless people die earlier than the rest of the population – that is, homelessness is associated with higher mortality.

Services can adopt an outreach approach; this is an effective strategy in reaching and targeting 'hard-to-reach' populations, providing a service that is accessible and flexible in approach. While outreach is important and valuable, it is just as important to ensure that centre-based services are designed in such a way that they can accommodate the 'hard-to reach'. Those providing wound services should commit themselves to establishing imaginative and innovative responses to meet the needs of this vulnerable group.

Fair access to primary and secondary care for some people in the UK remains problematic. The experiences of people from hard-to-reach groups offer important insights into barriers to accessing care. There is a need to provide local care that is pluralistic, adaptive and holistic, in order to ensure that there is equitable access to wound care services.

Appropriate dressing choice and skilled wound management are certainly essential aspects of wound healing; there are a number of other physical and psychosocial factors that are equally important. At the heart of effective healthcare provision is a successful therapeutic relationship between practitioners and patients.

48 Malignant wounds and palliative wound care

Figure 48.1 Fungating malignant breast wound.

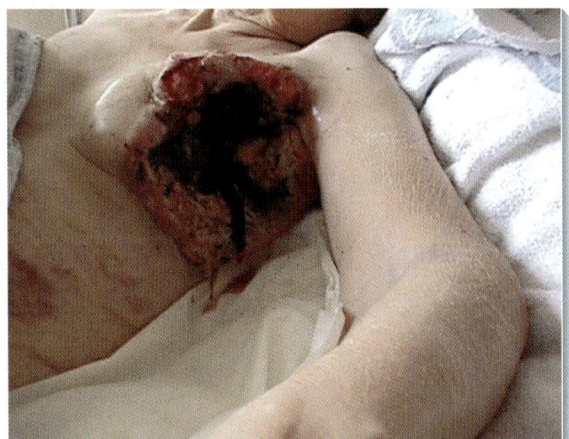

Figure 48.2 Fungating leg ulcer.

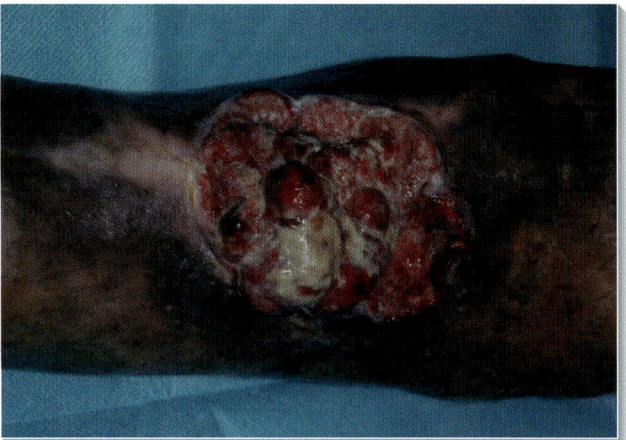

Source: Onesti et al 2013, figure 4a, p. 3. Reproduced with permission of John Wiley & Sons, Ltd.

Figure 48.3 Early-stage malignant wound, often mistaken for hypergranulation tissue.

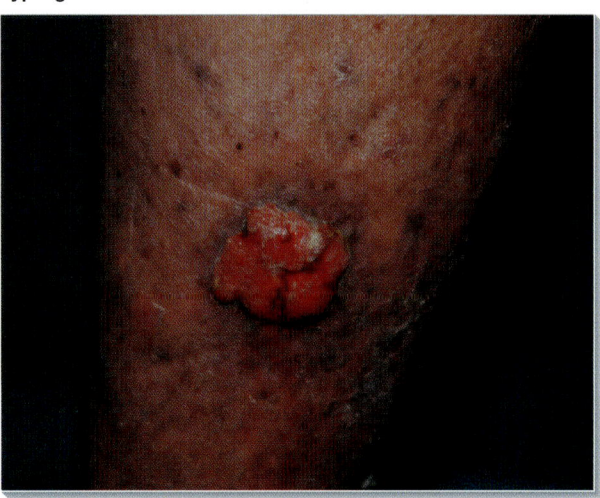

Source: Onesti et al 2013, figure 2, p. 2. Reproduced with permission of John Wiley & Sons, Ltd.

Wound Care at a Glance, Second Edition. Ian Peate and Melanie Stephens.
© 2020 John Wiley & Sons Ltd. Published 2020 by John Wiley & Sons Ltd.
Companion website: http://www.ataglanceseries.com/nursing/woundcare/

Malignant wounds are also known as malignant tumours, fungating ulcers, cancerous wounds or ulcerating wounds. The description of a fungating ulcer is derived from the appearance of the wound that grows in the shape of a fungus or a cauliflower (Figures 48.1 and 48.2). Most malignant wounds develop in cancers that affect the breast, head, neck, skin and groin or anal areas, but can also occur anywhere on the body. Unless the cancer is eradicated, these wounds fail to heal, and so the aim of care is to maintain an optimum control of the symptoms these wounds can produce, such as malodour, high levels of exudate and increased levels of pain, while protecting the surrounding skin from additional damage from poor wound care techniques and choices.

Why malignant wounds occur

Malignant wounds occur when an underlying disease (cancer) causes a wound to erupt through the skin. Sometimes, the malignancy starts in the epithelial cells of the body to form a wound. The malignancy may be of a primary origin (where the cancer originates) or can be spread from other parts of the body to form a new, secondary cancer on another part of the body and may or may not produce a wound. In any event, a medical diagnosis is required to determine whether or not any wound on a cancer patient is related to the malignancy.

In many cases, it is the wound itself that raises suspicion of malignancy; for example, when a patient who has no previous diagnosis of cancer has a wound that fails to heal, a nurse may suspect malignancy and can request a biopsy that can confirm the diagnosis.

Suspecting a malignant wound

In these cases, it is common for the patient to be cared for by a nurse for wound dressings for many months and even years without any significant healing rate. This is because the underlying cause (i.e. cancer) is not identified and addressed, making the wound unable to heal.

Unless the nurse is aware of the common signs associated with these wound types, the patient's condition continues to be left untreated, to the patient's detriment. A wound of significant longevity that fails to heal must therefore be referred to and reassessed by a specialist for further investigations. This could be referred to a tissue viability nurse or a doctor in the first instance, and then to a dermatologist for wound biopsy or other investigations. It is common practice to refer any patient with a wound that fails to heal, or progress towards healing within 6 weeks, to a tissue viability nurse or a doctor. In that time, the nurse is expected to adhere to the best practices in wound management, as described in this book. If the nurse is highly suspicious of malignancy in a wound before this time, it is wise to make this referral sooner than the aforementioned 6-week timeframe.

Common signs of a malignant wound

The most suspicious signs are the lack of identifiable causes and the wound's failure to heal. The malignant wound is often very perfectly round in shape; the tissue on the wound bed often alters shape and size very quickly (from one day to the next), and is often mistaken for hypergranulating tissue (discussed in other chapters) (Figure 48.3), not least due to its cauliflower appearance and friable tissue that bleeds easily. The wound is often painless and/or itchy. Occasionally, a wound may heal and then recur again in a cyclical manner. These symptoms do not confirm a malignant wound but, should raise the suspicions of the assessing nurse.

As the disease within the wound progresses, the symptoms become more obvious in terms of increased exudate levels – a more profound, larger wound with tissue that sits proud as compared to the surrounding skin, with the wound often bleeding very easily. There may be a malodour and the patient may complain of increasing pain or loss of function, particularly on a limb. Lymphoedema may occur, as can be seen in Figure 48.1. Prompt referral and diagnosis are essential in these cases.

Management of the malignant wound

First and foremost, a medical diagnosis is required to determine whether or not the wound is malignant. In some cases, the patient can be treated to eliminate the cancer; this can include radiotherapy, chemotherapy or surgery for short-term symptom relief. However, in many cases, there is no treatment available, and it is the nurse's responsibility to monitor and manage the symptoms sufficiently to enable the patient to achieve an optimum quality of life. This is known as 'palliative wound care'.

Palliative wound care

'Palliative care' is a term used when a patient's disease is no longer responsive to treatments, and the condition is rendering the patient more and more debilitated as he/she approaches the end of the life. Patients in this situation often either have existing wounds as a result of their terminal condition (e.g. surgical wounds or fungating ulcers), or they develop wounds (e.g. pressure ulcers and skin tears) as a result of their declining general health. By nature of the underlying causative disease, they are likely to have significant pain levels to deal with, and the presence of a wound can add to those pain levels if not adequately managed. In many cases of palliative care, it is improbable that a wound heals, and chances are that it gets larger, and so the aim of treating wounds in these patients changes from promoting healing to managing and controlling the symptoms associated with wounds, and, as far as possible, preventing deterioration. That is not to say our aims should not include creating the right wound conditions that would promote healing if it were possible, but simply states that our priorities and expectations must change for the sake of the patient's comfort and quality of life. Many wounds heal in the end-of-life stages with appropriate wound management. However, inappropriate wound management could hasten the death of the patient and is unacceptable.

Priorities in wound care: management of symptoms

As always, a nursing priority is to assess the patient holistically, taking into consideration the physical, psychological, emotional, environmental and social aspects affecting the patient. In particular, consideration must be given to the patient's nutritional status, mobility, site of the wound and the patients (substantial) potential for infection, as well as assessing the pain levels experienced by the patient in order to prescribe treatments that will meet their needs while minimising or reducing the patient's pain.

Exudate management: All wounds produce exudate, and malignant wounds are no exception. Indeed, this type of wound often produces excessive amounts of exudate due to the underlying destruction of lymph glands and other underlying tissues, making the wound the easiest route for the escape of other bodily fluids. As the exudate levels increase, bacteria are provided with an optimum environment to multiply in, and so the exudate levels increase and the cycle continues. Patients often become isolated because they fear the embarrassment of exudate leakage when they are in the company of others. The dressings used to manage exudate in malignant wounds should provide: a moist and warm environment to prevent the dressing sticking to the wound bed; capacity to absorb the levels of exudate produced by the malignancy; high-moisture vapour transfer; and conform and fit both the site and size of the wound. The amount and colour of exudate should be assessed, as these may be the first signs of an underlying infection. Secondary dressings that are highly absorbent or wound manager bags can assist with managing high levels of exudate. The surrounding skin should also be protected with skin barrier products to reduce the risk of excoriation or maceration. Referral to a dietician may be required if exudate production is high, as it can lead to protein depletion.

Malodour: It occurs as a result of increased bacterial growth, necrotic tissue and stale exudate. The higher the levels of bacteria, especially anaerobic bacteria, the greater the malodour is, due to the release of volatile fatty acids. This can have devastating impact on the patient, causing symptoms of nausea, gagging, reduced appetite, weight loss and social isolation. Dressings containing active charcoal or antimicrobials can be used. However, once a charcoal dressing becomes wet, it loses its odour absorbing properties and should be changed. Other methods to reduce odour from a malignant wound are drops of perfume or essential oils on clothing, and the use of deodorisers around the home.

Pain: Many malignant wounds are very painful for the patient and effective assessment and monitoring of pain levels and efficacy of analgesics are crucial to promote an acceptable pain level for the patient. Pain can be exacerbated by inappropriate and ineffectual exudate management, as bacteria and fungus rapidly increase in a wet environment. The waste products from the bacteria alter the pH value within the exudate, making the tissues (and nerve endings) more sensitive as a result of this change in environment. Different types of pain require different methods of management. Cutaneous pain can be soothed with the use of topical analgesia, prescribed and managed by the GP or palliative care team. Pain at dressing changes can be managed with short-acting pre-planned analgesia. Non-adherent or low-adherent dressings as a contact layer reduce discomfort on removal. The nursing team may even refer the patient for complementary therapies, such as visualisation, distraction and relaxation. If the pain is unmanaged, referral to the pain team or services can be necessary.

Infection: As stated earlier, malignant wounds can become heavily colonised or infected with bacteria. As the wound cannot be healed and the blood supply to the wound is generally impaired, systemic antibiotics to treat the infection are sometimes ineffective. If the wound is clinically infected, signs and symptoms such as erythema, induration, increased pain and exudate, leucocytosis and fever should be apparent. A wound swab should be taken, and topical antibiotics such as metronidazole (applied daily) can be considered. However, its effectiveness at treating the infection depends on whether there is a lot of necrosis and exudate at the wound bed. Other methods to reduce the number of bacteria at the wound bed include wound-cleansing products containing polyhexamethylene biguanide (PHMB) and/or antimicrobial dressings.

Itching: It can become an ongoing issue for patients with malignant wounds, as their skin is often stretched and nerve endings are irritated. Attention to good levels of hygiene to the peri-wound area and skin barrier products to protect, soothe and relieve the skin may be required.

Bleeding: Bleeding at the wound bed is a constant worry for patients, their significant others and healthcare professionals. Discussions about this with the patient and carers must be handled with sensitivity and care, especially around the associated risks and advanced decision-making.

As friable blood vessels and erosion of blood vessels from necrosis, sloughing, trauma and friction can lead to major haemorrhage, a risk assessment should be carried out. This includes examining for signs of visible pulsations in malignant wounds, frequent small episodes of bleeding, a sudden increase in pain, the patient taking anticoagulants or clotting abnormalities, site of the cancer and coexisting disease.

Control of the bleeding can be through applying direct local pressure to the area; however, this should be with caution so as not to cause pain. Alginate dressings can be applied to assist with haemostasis with small bleeds. The nurse should consider using a non-adherent primary contact layer to reduce the number of dressing changes and risk of further trauma and bleeding. If there is a large bleed that does not cease, a referral to a surgeon for cautery may be required. This would be considered an emergency and requires immediate medical attention, unless the patient has an advanced care plan and the decision is to remain at home.

Wound cleansing: This is only required when there is excess exudate, pus or serous fluid. This is because cleansing may increase the risk of trauma, bleeding and pain. If wound cleansing is required, the fluid should be warmed. The type of solution used depends on the presence of bacteria (heavily colonised or infected), the site of the malignant wound and if bone is visible. Some wounds may be cleansed with warm water whilst showering (soap must not come in contact with the wound); others may require an aseptic non-touch technique (if bone is visible) or clean technique.

Debridement: This should not be commenced unless directed by a tissue viability specialist or consultant due to the risk of bleeding. If the wound bed is filled with necrosis that is dry and the patient's prognosis is poor, the management may be to keep the wound dry, managing any odour and pain. This is because introducing moisture leads to high levels of exudate, increasing the risk of infection and malodour.

Psychological care: Patients with a malignant wound have a constant reminder of their diagnosis, prognosis and mortality. Symptoms of pain, malodour, exudate and itching can lead to embarrassment and social isolation. The nurse should not only address wound symptoms, but psychological ones too, referring patients for other coping therapies too.

Pressure ulcer prevention: As the skin is the first organ to fail in palliative and end-of-life patients, this may lead to the development or deterioration of pressure ulcers. This does not mean that worsening of the skin should be accepted as a norm, and a useful mnemonic 'Skin Changes At Life's End' (SCALE, 2009) can be used to guide practice. In the terminally ill patient, care must be carefully planned in conjunction with the patient, so that a repositioning interval can be agreed that is within the patient's individual tolerance level, and the most suitable pressure redistributing devices can be used to adequately achieve the agreed repositioning regimen. Very small, frequent position changes can be acceptable to patients rather than one complete change from one side to the other every 2 hours or so. This can be achieved by moving the patient gradually at smaller angles and at shorter intervals from one side to the other until the patient reaches the 30° tilt on one side and then the other. If done in conjunction with appropriate equipment (e.g. a low-air-loss mattress and a profiling bed), this may be acceptable to the patient and may minimise the risk of pressure ulcer development. However, in many cases, pressure damage occurs despite the best efforts, due to the failing nature of the patient's general health, and particularly if the patient is unable to tolerate such a repositioning regimen.

Glossary

Abrasion A wearing away of the skin through some mechanical process, such as friction or trauma
Abscess A circumscribed collection of pus that forms in tissue as a result of acute or chronic localised infection and is associated with tissue destruction and, in many cases, swelling
Acute wound Any wound that is new or progressing as expected
Alginate A non-woven, highly absorptive dressing that is manufactured from seaweed (kelp)
Angiogenesis The formation and regeneration of blood vessels
Antimicrobial An agent that kills microbes or inhibits their growth
Autolysis The breakdown of tissues or cells by the body's own mechanisms, such as enzymes or white blood cells
Bacteria One-celled microorganisms that break down dead tissue; they have no true nucleus and reproduce by cell division
Blanchable erythema A reddened area of the skin that temporarily turns white or pale when pressure is applied with a fingertip
Burn An acute wound caused by exposure to thermal extremes, electricity, radiation or caustic chemicals
Cellulitis An infection of the deeper layers of the skin and the underlying tissue
Chemical debridement Application, topically, of biological enzymes to break down devitalised tissue
Chronic wound A wound where healing is slow or stopped and it does not heal in a timely fashion
Collagen A supportive protein of skin, bone, tendon, connective tissue and cartilage
Colonised A wound contaminated with bacteria
Debridement Removal of necrotic tissue providing the underlying healthy tissue to regenerate
Debris The remains of damaged cells or tissues
Dehiscence Complication of wound healing where the wound may fully or partially open up
Dermis The inner thick layer of the skin
Diabetic foot ulcer Localised injury to the skin and/or underlying tissue, below the ankle, in a person with diabetes
Enzyme A protein that acts as a catalyst, causing chemical changes to occur
Epidermis The skin's outermost layer
Epithelisation Regeneration of skin across the surface of a wound
Erythema Redness of the skin caused by engorgement of the capillaries
Eschar Dead wound tissue appearing as a dry, leathery crust
Evisceration The protrusion of a visceral organ from a wound
Excoriation Skin abrasions
Exudate Any fluid that filters from the circulatory system into lesions or areas of inflammation
Fascia A layer of fibrous tissue
Fibrin An insoluble protein formed from fibrinogen during the clotting of blood, forming a fibrous mesh, impeding the flow of blood
Fibroblasts A type of cell that synthesises the extracellular matrix and collagen, the structural framework for tissues, and plays a central role in healing wounds; fibroblasts are the most common cells of connective tissue
Full-thickness wound A wound penetrating completely through the skin, protruding through the underlying tissues; bone may be exposed
Granulation Occurs where new connective tissue and tiny blood vessels form on the surfaces of a wound during the healing process; typically, granulation tissue grows from the base of a wound and is able to fill almost any size of wound

Hydrocolloid A wafer type of dressing containing gel-forming agents in an adhesive compound laminated onto a flexible, water-resistant outer layer; some types include an alginate to increase absorption capabilities
Hydrogel A water-based non-adherent type of dressing with some ability to absorb
Hydrophilic Has the ability to attract water – readily absorbs moisture
Hypoxia Reduction in the amount of oxygen reaching the tissues
Induration A process where the skin becomes firm; often surrounds a wound as a healing ridge
Incontinence The unwanted and involuntary leakage of urine or stool
Inflammation This is a localised protective response that causes heat, redness, swelling, pain and loss of function; during this phase, the body attempts to close off broken blood vessels and clean up the wound
Ischaemia A deficiency of blood supply to an area
Keloid A type of scar that is often red and prominent; it is caused by excessive collagen formation in the corium during connective tissue repair
Keratin An insoluble protein forming the principal component of epidermis, hair, nails and tooth enamel
Leg ulcer A chronic wound that takes more than 4–6 weeks to heal; develops on the inside of the leg, just above the ankle
Leucocytes The colourless blood corpuscles whose chief function is to protect the body against micro-organisms
Lymphocyte A mononuclear, non-granular leucocyte, chiefly a product of lymphoid tissue, which participates in the immune response
Lymphoedema A swelling that develops as a result of an impaired lymphatic system
Maceration A softening and whitish look to the intact skin around wounds caused by excessive moisture; often occurs when exudate is not well managed by dressings
Macrophage Any of the large, mononuclear, phagocytotic cells derived from monocytes that are found in the walls of blood vessels and in loose connective tissue; they become stimulated by inflammation on initial angiogenesis
Matrix The intracellular substance of a tissue that forms the framework of tissues
Maturation A phase in wound healing where scar tissue is remodelled
Mechanical debridement The removal of dead or devitalised tissue by use of wet to dry dressings, whirlpool, lavage or scrubbing (e.g. with gauze)
Myofibroblast A differentiated fibroblast containing the ultrastructural features of a fibroblast and a smooth muscle cell containing many actin-rich microfilaments
Necrosis Death of tissue or cell
Neutrophil White blood cell responsible for phagocytosis
Non-blanching erythema Redness of the skin persisting when gentle pressure is applied and then released
Occlusive dressing A dressing that closes the wound from the external environment
Pathogen An organism that can cause disease, such as a virus, bacteria or other micro-organism
Phagocytosis The process where cells surround and digest cell debris, micro-organisms, necrotic tissue and foreign bodies
Pressure ulcer A localised injury to the skin and/or underlying tissue, usually over a bony prominence, as a result of pressure, or pressure in combination with shear

Wound Care at a Glance, Second Edition. Ian Peate and Melanie Stephens.
© 2020 John Wiley & Sons Ltd. Published 2020 by John Wiley & Sons Ltd.
Companion website: http://www.ataglanceseries.com/nursing/woundcare/

Proliferation The growth or reproduction of tissue as part of the healing process
Pus A thick, yellowish fluid composed of dead bacteria and leucocytes
Purulent Containing or pus-forming
Scab Dry crust forming over an open wound; consists of skin and debris
Septicaemia Blood poisoning, a systemic disease where pathogenic micro-organisms are present and multiply in the blood
Slough Dead tissue, often yellow in colour; can be stringy in appearance
Suppuration Formation of discharge or pus
Suture A stitch or series of stitches made to secure the opposition of the edges of a surgical or traumatic wound
Tensile strength The strength of a closed or healed wound in terms of the greatest stress the tissues can bear without tearing
Wound Any break in the skin
Wound assessment An element of wound management that collects holistic information about the patient and the wound before a treatment plan is prescribed

References and further reading

BAPEN (2018). The MUST toolkit. https://www.bapen.org.uk/screening-and-must/must/must-toolkit/the-must-itself. Last accessed February 2019.

Baranoski, S. and Ayello, E.A. (2016). *Wound Care Essential. Practice Principles*, 4th Ed. Philadelphia: Wolters Kluwer.

Benbow, M. (2016). Best practice in wound assessment. *Nursing Standard* 30(27): 40–47.

Bergstrom, N. (1987). The Braden Scale for predicting pressure sore risk. *Nurse Researcher* 36(4): 205–210.

Brown, A. (2015). Wound Management 3: The assessment and treatment of wound pain. *Nursing Times* 111(47): 15–17.

Bryant, R.A. (2016). *Acute and Chronic Wounds. Current Management Concepts*, 5th Ed. Elsevier: St Louis.

Chamanga, E.T. (2018). Clinical management of non-healing wounds. *Nursing Standard* 32(29): 48–62.

Coleman, S., Nelson, E.A., Keen, J. et al. (2014). Developing a pressure ulcer risk factor minimum data set and risk assessment framework. *Journal of Advanced Nursing* 70(10): 2339–2352.

Crane, M.A., Caetano, G., Joly, L.M. et al. (2018). *Mapping of Specialist Primary Health Care Services in England for People who are Homeless*. London: Social Care Workforce Research Unit King's College.

European Pressure Ulcer Advisory Panel, National Pressure Ulcer Advisory Panel & the Pan Pacific Pressure Injury Alliance (2014). Prevention and treatment of pressure ulcers: Quick reference guide. Retrieved from http://www.npuap.org/wp-content/uploads/2014/08/Quick-Reference-Guide-DIGITAL-NPUAP-EPUAP-PPPIA-Jan2016.pdf

European Wound Management Association (2008). Hard-to-heal wounds: A holistic approach. Retrieved 23 April 2019 from https://ewma.org/it/resources/for-professionals/ewma-documents-and-joint-publications/ewma-position-documents-2002-2008/

Falanga, V. (2004). *Wound Bed Preparation in Practice. EWMA Position Document*, pp. 2–5. London: Medical Education Partnership Ltd.

Fingeret, M.C., Teo, I. and Epner, D.E. (2014). Managing body image difficulties of adult cancer patients: Lessons from available research. *Cancer* 120(5 pp): 633–641. doi:10.1002/cncr.28469.

Flanagan, M. (2013). *Wound Healing and Skin Integrity: Principles and Practice*. Oxford: Wiley.

Glasper, A. and Rees, C. (2017). *Nursing and Healthcare Research At A Glance*. Oxford: Wiley.

Grove, S.K. and Burns, N. (2019). *Understanding Nursing Research: Building an Evidence-Based Practice*, 7th Ed. Elsevier. St Louis.

Guest, J.F., Ayoub, N., McIlwraith, T. et al. (2015). Health economic burden that wounds impose on the National Health Service in the UK. *BMJ Open* 5(12): e009283.

LeBlanc, K., Baranoski, S., Christensen, D. et al. (2013). International skin tear advisory panel (ISTAP) – Validation of a new classification system for skin tears. *Advances in Skin & Wound Care* 26(6): 263–265.

Lloyd-Jones, M. (2015). A short history of the development of wound care dressings. *British Journal of Healthcare Assistants* 9(10): 482–485.

McCance, K.L. and Heuther, S.E. (2018) *Pathophysiology: The Biologic Basis for Disease in Adults and Children*, 8th Ed. St Louis: Elsevier.

Migliozzi, J. (2018) Inflammation, immune response and healing. Ch 3 in *Fundamentals of Applied Pathophysiology. An Essential Guide for Nursing and Healthcare Students*, 3rd Ed. (ed. Peate, I.), 62–92. Oxford: Wiley.

National Institute of Health and Care Excellence (2019). Surgical site infections: Prevention and treatment. https://www.nice.org.uk/guidance/ng125/resources/surgical-site-infections-prevention-and-treatment-pdf-66141660564421. Last accessed July 2019.

National Institute for Health and Care Excellence (2016). Chronic wounds: Advanced wound dressings and antimicrobial dressings. https://www.nice.org.uk/advice/esmpb2/resources/chronic-wounds-advanced-wound-dressings-and-antimicrobial-dressings-pdf-1502609570376901. Last accessed February 2019.

National Institute of Health and Clinical Excellence (2015). Pressure ulcers. https://www.nice.org.uk/guidance/qs89/resources/pressure-ulcers-pdf-2098916972485. Last accessed February 2019.

National Institute of Health and Care Excellence (2014). Pressure ulcers: Prevention and management. Retrieved 24 April 2019 from http://www.nice.org.uk/guidance/cg179/chapter/1-recommendations

National Institute for Health and Care Excellence (2014). Anxiety disorders. https://www.nice.org.uk/guidance/qs53/resources/anxiety-disorders-pdf-2098725496261. Last accessed January 2019.

NHS Improvement (2018). Pressure ulcers: Revised definition and measurement: Summary and recommendations. Retrieved 24 April2019fromhttps://improvement.nhs.uk/resources/pressure-ulcers-revised-definition-and-measurement-framework/

Nixon, J., Nelson, E.A., Rutherford, C. et al. (2015). Pressure UlceR programme of reSEarch (PURPOSE): Using mixed methods (systematic reviews, prospective cohort, case study, consensus and psychometrics) to identify patient and organisational risk, develop a risk assessment tool and patient-reported outcome quality of life and health utility measures. https://www.ncbi.nlm.nih.gov/books/NBK321049/. Last accessed February 2019.

National Institute of Health and Care Excellence (2013). Varicose veins: Diagnosis and management (CG168). https://www.nice.org.uk/guidance/cg168/resources/varicose-veins-diagnosis-and-management-pdf-35109698485957. Last accessed February 2019.

National Institute for Health and Care Excellence (2012). Nutritional support in adults. https://www.nice.org.uk/guidance/qs24/chapter/quality-statement-1-screening-for-the-risk-of-malnutrition. Last accessed February 2019.

Nursing and Midwifery Council (2018). The code. Retrieved 23 April 2019 from https://www.nmc.org.uk/standards/code/read-the-code-online/

Peate, I. (2016). The skin. Ch 17 in *Fundamentals of Anatomy and Physiology for Nursing and Health Care Students*, 2nd Ed. (ed. Peate, I. and Nair, M.), 555–574. Oxford: Wiley.

Queen's Nursing Institute (2015). *Assessing the Health of People Who Are Homeless: Guidance with Health Assessment Tool*. London: QNI

Roper, N. (1988). *Principles of Nursing in Process Context*. Edinburgh: Churchill Livingstone.

Scottish Intercollegiate Guidelines Network (2010). Management of chronic venous leg ulcers. https://www.sign.ac.uk/assets/sign120.pdf. Last accessed February 2019.

Sibbald, R.G., Krasner, D.L. and Lutz, J. (2010). SCALE: Skin changes at life's end. Final consensus statement. *Advances in Skin & Wound Care*, 23(5): 225–236.

Stephens, M. (2018). The principles of skin integrity. Ch 18 in *Nursing Practice, Knowledge and Care*, 2nd Ed. (ed. Peate, I. and Wild, K.), 350– 375 Oxford: Wiley.

Stephens, M. and Bartley, C.A. (2017). Understanding the association between pressure ulcers and sitting in adults what does it mean for me and my carers? Seating guidelines for people, carers and health & social care professionals. *Journal of Tissue Viability*, 27(1): 59–73.

Tippett, A. (2011). Treat the patient, not the wound. https://www.woundsource.com/blog/treat-patient-not-wound. Last accessed February 2019.

Waugh, A. and Grant, A. (2018) *Ross and Wilson Anatomy and Physiology in Health and Illness*, 13th Ed. Edinburgh: Elsevier.

Williams, P. (2018). *deWit's Fundamental Concepts and Skills for Nursing*, 5th Ed. Elsevier: St Louis.

Winter, G.D. (1962). Formation of the scab and the rate of epithelialization of superficial wounds in the skin of young domestic pigs. *Nature* 193: 293–294.

Wisley, J. (2013). The impact of psychological distress on the healing of burns. *Wound UK* 9(Suppl. 3): 14–17.

World Health Organization (1986). *Cancer Pain Relief*. Geneva: World Health Press.

Wounds UK (2012). Best practice statement. *Care of the Older Person's Skin*, 2nd Ed. London: Wounds UK.

Useful resources: websites

British Burns Association. https://www.britishburnsassociation.org/

British National Formulary Online. https://www.bnf.org/products/bnf-online/

Diabetes UK Putting Feet First campaign. https://www.diabetes.org.uk/professionals/position-statements-reports/specialist-care-for-children-and-adults-and-complications/putting-feet-first-diabetes-foot-care

European Wound Management Association. https://ewma.org/

International Skin Tear Advisory Panel. http://www.skintears.org/

Legs Matter. https://legsmatter.org/

Lindsay Leg Club Foundation. www.legclub.org/about-us/leg-club-foundation

NHS Improvement (2018). Stop the pressure. Retrieved 23 April 2019 from http://nhs.stopthepressure.co.uk/

Nursing and Midwifery Council. https://www.nmc.org.uk/

Purpose T Resources. https://xforms.leeds.ac.uk/forms/form/465/en/accessing_purpose_t_and_pupps_resources

Waterlow Score. http://www.judy-waterlow.co.uk/waterlow_score.htm

Index

Page locators in **bold** indicate tables/boxes. Page locators in *italics* indicate figures. This index uses letter-by-letter alphabetization.

ABPI *see* ankle–brachial pressure index
abrasion *112*, 113
absorbent cellulose fibre gelling agents 73
activities of living (ALs) 51
acute wounds 15–25
   classification of wounds *46*, 47
   factors affecting wound-healing 24–25, *24*
   haemostasis 16–17, *16*
   inflammation 18–19, *18*
   maturation 21, 22–23, *22*
   proliferation, granulation, and epithelialisation 20–21, *20*
   wound assessment 43
adhesive strips *108*, 110
ALs *see* activities of living
age
   anatomy and physiology 12–13, **12**
   chronic wounds 30
   wounds in different populations 119
alcohol use 41
alginates **64**, 66
allergies 41
amputation 9
analgesic ladder *56*, 57
anatomy and physiology 1–13
   ageing skin 12–13, **12**
   body image 8–10, *8*, **8**
   history of wound care 2–3, **2**
   psychosocial aspects of the skin 6–7, *6*
   skin 4–5, *4*
ankle–brachial pressure index (ABPI)
   arterial leg ulcers 95
   assessing for arterial disease 96–98, *96*
   chronic wounds 37
   compression therapy 93
   interpreting ABPIs 100–101, **100**
   venous leg ulcers 89
antimicrobials and antibiotics
   dressings 66, 70–73, *70*
   history of wound care 3
anxiety 7
arterial leg ulcers
   chronic wounds *36*, 37
   classification of wounds *46*, 47
   complexities of wound care 94–95, *94*

arteriosclerosis 37, *94*, 95
aseptic technique 51, 60, 122
assessment tools 41
ASSKING care bundle 83–84
atypical wounds 116–117, *116*
autolytic debridement 55
avulsions 113

barrier creams/sprays 75, 107
biofilms 71
biphasic sounds 101
bites *112*, 113
blanching erythema 106
blastomycosis 117
bleeding 109
blood vessels 5
body image 8–10, *8*, **8**
bruising *112*, 113
Buerger's disease 37
Buerger's test 37
bullous pemphigoid *116*, 117
burns 114–115, *114*, **114**
   classification of wounds 47
   traumatic wounds 113

cadexomer iodine 73
capillary refill 37
carbohydrates 33
care planning 51, 61
cavity wounds 90, 109
CBT *see* cognitive behavioural therapy
cell-based therapies 77
cellulose fibre gelling agents 73
Changing Faces campaign poster 6
Charcot osteoarthropathy 103
chemical burns *114*, 115
chemokines, acute wounds 19
chronic wounds 27–37
   classification of wounds *46*, 47
   factors affecting wound-healing 30–31
   haemostasis 29
   impaired wound-healing 27–28, *27*
   incontinence 34–35, *34*, **34**
   inflammation 29
   intrinsic/extrinsic factors 29, 30
   maturation 29
   nutrition 30, 32–33, *32*
   regeneration 29
   vascular disease 36–37, *36*
   wound assessment 43
clean technique 51, 122

clotting cascade 16, 17, 19
cognitive behavioural therapy (CBT) 7
collagen 23
communication strategies **8**, 84
comorbidities 30, 87
complexities of wound care 79–123
   arterial leg ulcers 94–95, *94*
   assessing for arterial disease 96–98, *96*, **96**
   atypical wounds 116–117, *116*
   burns and scalds 113, 114–115, *114*, **114**
   compression therapy 89, 91, 92–93, *92*, **92**, 100, 101
   diabetic foot ulcers 102–104, *102*
   interpreting ABPIs 100–101, **100**
   lymphoedema 90–91, *90*
   malignant wounds and palliative wound care 120–123, *120*
   moisture lesions 82, 83, 106–107, *106*, **106**
   pressure redistribution equipment 80–81, *80*
   pressure ulcer classification and prevention 82–84, *82*
   pressure ulcers 86–87, *86*
   surgical wounds 108–110, *108*, **108**
   traumatic wounds 112–113, *112*, **112**
   venous leg ulcers 88–89, *88*
   wounds in different populations 118–119, *118*
comprehensive pain assessment *56*, 57
compression therapy
   complexities of wound care 92–93, *92*, **92**
   interpreting ABPIs **100**, 101
   lymphoedema 91
   venous leg ulcers 89
compression ultrasound 98
contusions 47, *112*, 113
creams
   application 74, 75
   lymphoedema 91
   moisture lesions 107
cutaneous tuberculosis *116*, 117
cuts *112*, 113
cytokines 23

DACC *see* dialkyl carbamoyl chloride
debridement 54, 55, 122
deep tissue injury *82*, 83
deep vein thrombosis (DVT) 98
dehiscence 109
delayed primary intention 55
deodorisers **64**, 65–66
dermis 5, 13
DFU *see* diabetic foot ulcers
diabetic foot ulcers (DFU) 30, 102–104, *102*
dialkyl carbamoyl chloride (DACC) 72
documenting wounds 50–51, *50*, 109
Doppler ultrasound
   arterial leg ulcers 95
   assessing for arterial disease 96, **96**, 97–98
   interpreting ABPIs 101
   vascular disease 37
   venous leg ulcers 89
dressings 59–77
   advanced technologies 76–77, *76*
   antimicrobials and antibiotics 66, 70–73, *70*
   application of lotions, creams, emollients and ointments 74–75, *74*
   aseptic technique 60
   care planning 61
   choosing a wound care product 68–69, *68*
   chronic wounds 30
   diabetic foot ulcers 104
   exudate 60, 62–63, *62*
   generic wound products: mode of action 64–66, **64–65**
   irrigation 60
   moisture lesions 107
   pain management 60
   swabs 60
   tissue, infection, moisture, time 68, 69
   venous leg ulcers 89
   wound management 60–61
   wounds in different populations 119
drug history 41
dry wound environment 62, 63, 68
DVT *see* deep vein thrombosis
dynamic alternating air mattress/cushion 80, 81

Wound Care at a Glance, Second Edition. Ian Peate and Melanie Stephens.
© 2020 John Wiley & Sons Ltd. Published 2020 by John Wiley & Sons Ltd.
Companion website: http://www.ataglanceseries.com/nursing/woundcare/

EBP *see* evidence-based practice
economical factors 25
electrical burns 113, 115
electrical stimulation 77
emollients 74, 75, 91
emotional factors 7, 9, 25
environmental factors 25, 30
enzyme alginogel 71
epidermis 5, 13
epithelialisation 20–21, 46, 47
ethical aspects 48–49, 48
evidence-based practice (EBP) 52–53, *52*, **52**
evisceration 109
excoriation 35, 107
extrinsic factors 29, 30
extrinsic pathway *16*, 17
exudate
    diabetic foot ulcers 104
    dressings 60, 62–63, *62*
    malignant wounds 121–122

fibrin meshwork *16*, 17
fistulas 109
foams **64**, 65
foot protectors *80*, 81
friction
    classification of wounds 47
    pressure ulcers 86, 87
    traumatic wounds *112*, 113
frostbite 113
fungating malignant wounds 9, *120*

gangrene *102*, 103–104
gas gangrene 103
gender 30
general health assessment 43
granulation
    acute wounds 20–21, *20*
    classification of wounds 46, 47
    hypergranulation 117

haemostasis 16–17, *16*, 29
hair 4, 5, 13
hierarchy of evidence **52**, 53
history of wound care 2–3, *2*
holistic assessment *24*, 25, 31
homelessness *118*, 119
honey/honey-impregnated dressings 71
hydration 33, 35
hydrocolloid 3, **64**, 65
hydrofibrous dressings **64**, 66
hydrogels/hydrogel sheet **65**, 66
hypergranulation 117
hypodermis 5

incisions 47, *112*, 113
incontinence
    chronic wounds 34–35, *34*, **34**
    pressure ulcers 83, 87
infection
    antimicrobials and antibiotics 66, 70–73, *70*
    classification of wounds 46, 47
    diabetic foot ulcers *102*, 103–104
    dressings 60, 68, 69
    malignant wounds 122

surgical wounds 109
    traumatic wounds 113
    wound management 44
inflammation
    acute wounds 18–19, *18*
    chronic wounds 29
    dressings 68
    wound management 44
intrinsic factors 29, 30
intrinsic pathway *16*, 17
iodine/iodine-impregnated dressings 72
irrigation 60, 109–110
ISTAP *see* International Skin Tear Advisory Panel
itching 122

keratinocytes 21

lacerations
    classification of wounds 46, 47
    traumatic wounds *112*, 113
Laplace's law *92*, 93
larval therapy 54, 55
    diabetic foot ulcers *102*
    dressings 76, 77
legal aspects 48–49, *48*
lifestyle 30, 41, 43
limb plethysmography 98
lotions *74*, 75
low-adherent dressings **65**, 66
low-air-loss devices 81
lymphatic system 5, 91
lymphoedema 90–91, *90*

maceration 35, 107
maggots *see* larval therapy
malignant wounds 120–123, *120*
    aetiology 121
    fungating malignant wounds 9, *120*
    palliative wound care 121
    wound assessment 121
    wound management 121–123
Malnutrition Universal Screening Tool (MUST) *32*, 33, 41, 84
malodour 122
mastectomy 9
maturation
    acute wounds 21, 22–23, *22*
    chronic wounds 29
MDFT *see* multidisciplinary diabetic foot team
medications 30, 87
mental health 119
methicillin-resistant *Staphylococcus aureus* (MRSA) 77
minerals 33
moist/damp wound environment
    diabetic foot ulcers 104
    dressings 61, *62*, 63, 68, 69
    pressure ulcers 87
    wound management 44
moisture lesions
    chronic wounds 34, **34**, 35
    complexities of wound care 106–107, *106*, **106**
    pressure ulcers 82, 83, **106**
moisturisers 75

monophasic sounds 101
MRSA *see* methicillin-resistant *Staphylococcus aureus*
multidisciplinary diabetic foot team (MDFT) 103
MUST *see* Malnutrition Universal Screening Tool

nails 4, 5, 13
National Institute for Health and Care Excellence (NICE) 87
necrosis
    classification of wounds 46, 47
    diabetic foot ulcers *102*, 103–104
negative pressure wound therapy 54, 55, 76, 77
nerve fibres 5
neuropathic foot ulcers *102*, 103
NHS Scotland Wound Assessment Chart *50*
NICE *see* National Institute for Health and Care Excellence
NMC *see* Nursing and Midwifery Council
non-blanching erythema 106
NOPQRST mnemonic **56**, 57
Nursing and Midwifery Council (NMC) 49
nursing process *42*, 44, 51
nutrition
    chronic wounds 30, 32–33, *32*
    pressure ulcers 84, 87

octenidine solution/cream/gel 72
ointments *74*, 75
overweight/obesity 91

PAD *see* peripheral artery disease
pain
    holistic approach 57
    malignant wounds 122
    pain assessment *56*, 57
    pain management 56–57, *56*, **56**, 60
    wound-related pain 57
palliative wound care 121
paper strip dressings *108*, 110
past medical history 41
patient history *40*, 41
PDGF *see* platelet derived growth factor
penetrating wounds *112*, 113
peripheral artery disease (PAD) 30, 95, 98, 101
person-centred therapy 93
phagocytosis 19
PHMB *see* polyhexamethylene biguanide
physical activity 89, 91
physical assessment 41
physical factors 25, 30
platelet derived growth factor (PDGF) 23
platelets 16, 17, 19
plethysmography 98
polyhexamethylene biguanide (PHMB) 72
povidone iodine 73
pressure redistribution equipment 80–81, *80*

pressure ulcers
    aetiology and additional causes 86, 87
    assessing for arterial disease 98
    chronic wounds 34, **34**, 35
    classification and prevention 82–84, *82*
    classification of wounds 47
    complexities of wound care 86–87, *86*
    diabetic foot ulcers *102*, 103
    dressings 69
    malignant wounds 122–123
    moisture lesions 82, 83, **106**
    risk assessment 87
    wound management 41
primary intention 54, 55
professional standards 49
proliferation 20–21, *20*
proteins 33
psychosocial factors
    anatomy and physiology 6–7, *6*
    body image 9
    holistic assessment 25
    malignant wounds 122
pulse 36, 37
pulse oximetry 98
puncture wounds 47, *112*, 113
PURPOSE-T assessment tool 87
pyoderma gangrenosum 117

record-keeping 50–51, *50*, 109
referral
    body image 10
    burns and scalds 115
    interpreting ABPIs 101
    psychosocial aspects of the skin 7
regeneration 29
remodelling 21
rheumatoid arthritis 30
rubor of dependency 37
rule of nines *114*, **114**

scalds 114–115, *114*, **114**
    classification of wounds 47
    traumatic wounds 113
scarring 7
scleroderma 117
sebaceous glands 4, 5
secondary intention 54, 55
self-esteem 8
sharp debridement 55
shearing 47, 86, 87
silver-impregnated dressings 72
skin
    ageing skin 12–13, **12**
    anatomy and physiology 4–5, *4*
    assessment 40–41, *40*
    pressure ulcers 83
    psychosocial aspects 6–7, *6*
skin tears 47, **112**, 113
sloughing
    classification of wounds 46, 47
    diabetic foot ulcers *102*, 104
smoking 41
staples *108*, 110
static foam mattress/cushion *80*, 81

129

steroid creams and lotions 75
Stigma Scale 10
stratum basale 5
stratum corneum 5
stratum granulosum 5
stratum lucidum 5
stratum spinosum 5
stress 7
structured wound assessment 42, 43–44
subcutaneous tissue 13
sunburn *114*
supporting wedges *80*, 81
surgical debridement *54*, 55
surgical wounds 108–110, *108*, **108**
   complications 109–110
   pre-, intra- and post-operative care 109
   removal of closure and dressing 110
suspected deep tissue injury *82*, 83
sutures *108*, 110
swabs 60
sweating 87

TBPI *see* toe–brachial pressure index
TBSA *see* total body surface area
temperature effects 30
tertiary intention 55

TGFβ *see* transforming growth factor-β
therapeutic relationship 119
tilt-in-place wheelchairs and chairs 81
tissue-based therapies 77
tissue viability
   documenting wounds and keeping records 51
   dressings 68, 69
   legal and ethical aspects 49
   wound management 44
TNFα *see* tumour necrosis factor-α
TNP *see* total negative pressure
toe–brachial pressure index (TBPI) *96*, **96**, 98
topical antimicrobials/antibiotics 71–73, 74–75, *74*
total body surface area (TBSA) 115
total negative pressure (TNP) *54*, 55, *76*, 77
transforming growth factor-β (TGFβ) 23
traumatic wounds 112–113, *112*, **112**
triphasic sounds 101
tumour necrosis factor-α (TNFα) 23

ulcerative colitis 30

vacuum-assisted closure (VAC) *54*, 55, *76*, 77
vascular disease 36–37, *36*
venous insufficiency 89
venous leg ulcers
   classification of wounds *46*, 47
   complexities of wound care 88–89, *88*
Versajet *76*, 77
visual analogue scales *56*, 57
vitamins 33

water/fluids 33, 35
wet wound environment *62*, 63
WHO analgesic ladder *56*, 57
wound assessment
   acute wounds 24–25, *24*
   body image 9–10
   chronic wounds 29, 31
   diabetic foot ulcers 103
   documenting wounds and keeping records 51
   frequency of assessment/nursing process *42*, 44, 51
   malignant wounds 121
   pressure ulcers 87
   structured wound assessment *42*, 43–44
   wound bed preparation 44
   wound management 42–44, *42*

wound bed preparation (WBP) 44, 68
wound closure
   primary intention *54*, 55
   secondary intention *54*, 55
   surgical wounds *108*, **108**, 109–110
wound edges 44, *68*, 69
wound management 39–57
   arterial leg ulcers 95
   assessment of skin 40–41, *40*
   atypical wounds 117
   burns and scalds 115
   chronic wounds 30
   classification of wounds 46–47, *46*
   documenting wounds and keeping records 50–51, *50*
   dressings 60–61
   evidence-based practice 52–53, *52*, **52**
   legal and ethical aspects 48–49, *48*
   lymphoedema 91
   malignant wounds 121–123
   pain management 56–57, *56*, **56**
   patient history *40*, 41
   treatment options 54–55, *54*
   wound assessment 42–44, *42*